Fire Safety and R[...]
Management Re[...]

The *Fire Safety and Risk Management Revision Guide: for the NEBOSH National Fire Certificate* is the perfect revision aid for students preparing to take their NEBOSH National Certificate in Fire Safety and Risk Management. As well as being a handy companion volume to the Fire Protection Association textbook *Fire Safety and Risk Management: for the NEBOSH National Certificate in Fire Safety and Risk Management*, it will also serve as a useful *aide-mémoire* for those in fire safety roles. The book:

▶ provides practical revision guidance and strategies for students;
▶ highlights the key information for each learning outcome of the current NEBOSH syllabus;
▶ gives students opportunities to test their knowledge based on NEBOSH-style questions and additional exercises;
▶ provides details of publically available guidance documents that students will be able to refer to.

The revision guide is fully aligned to the current NEBOSH syllabus, providing complete coverage in bite-sized chunks, helping students to learn and memorise the most important topics. Throughout the book, the guide refers to the *Fire Safety and Risk Management* textbook, helping students to consolidate their learning.

Jonathan Backhouse MRes MA BA (Hons) CertEd CMIOSH is a highly qualified teacher and Chartered Safety and Health Practitioner. Since becoming self-employed in 2002 he has gained a vast amount of health and safety experience, working as a consultant, trainer, assessor, examiner and author; working in the UK, Africa, Europe, the Middle East and the USA.

Ed Ferrett is former Vice Chairman of NEBOSH (1999–2008) and a lecturer on NEBOSH courses with both public and private course providers. He is a chartered engineer and health and safety consultant.

Fire Safety and Risk Management Revision Guide

For the NEBOSH National Fire Certificate

Jonathan Backhouse and Ed Ferrett

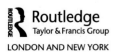

Routledge
Taylor & Francis Group

LONDON AND NEW YORK

First published 2017
by Routledge
2 Park Square, Milton Park, Abingdon, Oxon OX14 4RN

and by Routledge
711 Third Avenue, New York, NY 10017

Routledge is an imprint of the Taylor & Francis Group, an informa business

British Library Cataloguing in Publication Data
A catalogue record for this book is available from the British Library.

Library of Congress Cataloging in Publication Data
Names: Backhouse, Jonathan, author. | Ferrett, Ed, author.
Title: Fire safety and risk management revision guide for the NEBOSH national fire certificate / Jonathan Backhouse and Ed Ferrett.
Description: Abingdon, Oxon : Routledge, 2017. | Includes bibliographical references.
Identifiers: LCCN 2016028773 | ISBN 9781138230026 (hardback) | ISBN 9781138677739 (pbk.) | ISBN 9781315559360 (ebook)
Subjects: LCSH: Fire protection engineering—Examinations—Study guides. | Industrial safety—Examinations—Study guides. | National Examination Board in Occupational Safety and Health—Examinations—Study guides.
Classification: LCC TH9157 .B335 2017 | DDC 363.37—dc23
LC record available at https://lccn.loc.gov/2016028773

ISBN: 978-1-138-23002-6 (hbk)
ISBN: 978-1-138-67773-9 (pbk)
ISBN: 978-1-315-55936-0 (ebk)

Typeset in Univers
by Apex CoVantage, LLC
Printed and bound by CPI Group (UK) Ltd, Croydon, CR0 4YY

Contents

Preface

Welcome to the latest revision guide for the *NEBOSH National Certificate in Fire Safety and Risk Management*. The guide has been designed to be used together with the latest NEBOSH National Certificate in Fire Safety and Risk Management syllabus guide and the two textbooks, *Introduction to Health and Safety at Work* by Hughes and Ferrett (for NGC1) and *Fire Safety and Risk Management: for the NEBOSH National Certificate in Fire Safety and Risk Management* by the Fire Protection Association (for FC1). The guide gives only a basic summary of the NEBOSH National Certificate in Fire Safety and Risk Management course, and a full explanation of all the topics is given in the relevant textbook.

The revision guide has the following features:

▶ It follows the latest NEBOSH National Certificate in Fire Safety and Risk Management syllabus.
▶ Revision notes are included for each of the elements of the two units – NGC1 (Management of Health and Safety) and FC1: Fire safety and risk management.
▶ A summary of the learning outcomes and key points is given for each element.
▶ Important diagrams are included to help revision.
▶ The fire certificate (FC1) section of the guide includes revision questions and revision hints.

The revision guide will also be useful to those who have specific health and safety responsibilities in their jobs and those who are studying other courses that include important health and safety elements – for example, courses in engineering, business studies, the health services, and retail and hotel management. The compact size of the revision guide ensures that it can be easily carried and used for revision at any time or place.

Good luck with your studies.

List of principal abbreviations

ACOP	Approved Code of Practice
CDM	Construction (Design and Management) Regulations
EPA	Environmental Protection Act 1990 (UK)
EU	European Union
HSE	Health and Safety Executive
HSG	Health and Safety Guidance
HSW Act	Health and Safety at Work etc. Act 1974 (UK)
INDG	Industry Guidance
ILO	International Labour Office
IOSH	Institution of Occupational Safety and Health
ISO	International Organization for Standardization
MHSWR	Management of Health and Safety at Work Regulations
NEBOSH	National Examination Board in Occupational Safety and Health
PPE	Personal Protective Equipment
RIDDOR	Reporting of Injuries, Diseases and Dangerous Occurrences Regulations
ROES	Representative(s) of Employee Safety
RP	Responsible Person
RPE	Respiratory Protective Equipment
RRFSO	Regulatory Reform Fire Safety Order (UK)

Unit NGC1

Management of health and safety

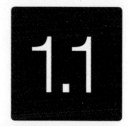

1.1

Foundations in health and safety

Learning outcomes

Outline the scope and nature of occupational health and safety ☐

Explain the moral, legal and financial reasons for promoting good standards of health and safety in the workplace ☐

Explain the legal framework for the regulation of health and safety, including sources and types of law ☐

Explain the scope, duties and offences of employers, managers, employees and others under the Health and Safety at Work etc. Act 1974 (HSW Act) ☐

Explain the scope, duties and offences of employers, managers, employees and others under the Management of Health and Safety at Work Regulations ☐

Outline the legal and organisational health and safety roles and responsibilities of clients and their contractor ☐

Outline the principles of assessing and managing contractors ☐

Unit NGC1 Management of health and safety

The definitions of hazard, risk, civil law, criminal law, common law and statute law ☐

The business case for health and safety (direct, indirect, insured and uninsured costs) ☐

The employer's duty of care and other common law and statutory duties ☐

Criminal offences and defences ☐

Civil liabilities and defences (particularly negligence) ☐

The legal framework – the Health and Safety at Work Act, the Management of Health and Safety at Work Regulations, absolute and qualified duties ☐

The powers of the enforcement officer, health and safety offences (including corporate manslaughter and corporate homicide), and penalties ☐

The role and functions of other external agencies ☐

The health and safety responsibilities and duties of employers to their employees and others affected by their undertaking, such as contractors, general public, visitors, patients and students ☐

The health and safety responsibilities of directors, managers, supervisors, employees and the self-employed ☐

Duties and responsibilities of manufacturers and others in the supply chain ☐

The duties and responsibilities between client and contractor to ensure a high standard of health and safety during the contract ☐

The legal duties under the Construction (Design and Management) Regulations ☐

The principles of selecting and managing contractors ☐

Definitions

▶ Accident – an unplanned event that results in damage, loss or harm
▶ Hazard – the potential of something to cause harm
▶ Risk – the likelihood of something to cause harm
▶ Civil law – duties of individuals to each other
▶ Criminal law – duties of individuals to the state
▶ Welfare – provision of facilities to maintain health and well-being of people in the workplace (e.g. washing, sanitary and first-aid)
▶ Residual risk – remaining risks after controls applied
▶ Near miss – any incident that could have resulted in an accident
▶ Dangerous occurrence – a near miss that could have led to serious injury or loss of life
▶ Common Law – law based on court judgments
▶ Statute Law – law based on Acts of Parliament.

Reasons for good health and safety management

Moral reasons

Need to provide a reasonable standard of care and ethical reasons to reduce:

▶ accident rates; and
▶ industrial disease and ill-health rates.

Legal reasons

Employers have a duty to take reasonable care of workers. Poor management can lead to:

▶ prosecutions; and
▶ civil actions – compensation claims.

Financial reasons

Poor health and safety management can lead to:

▶ direct costs; and
▶ indirect costs.

Good health and safety management can lead to:

▶ a more highly motivated workforce resulting in an improvement in the rate of production and product quality; and
▶ an improved image and reputation of the organisation with its various stakeholders.

Social reasons

These include:

▶ societal expectation of good standards of health and safety; and
▶ duty of care (details under 'Aspects of civil law' below).

Costs of accidents and ill-health

Direct costs

Directly related to the accident and may be insured or uninsured.

Insured direct costs normally include:

▶ claims on employers' and public liability insurance;
▶ damage to buildings, equipment or vehicles; and
▶ any attributable production and/or general business loss.

Uninsured direct costs include:

▶ fines resulting from prosecution by the enforcement authority;
▶ sick pay;
▶ some damage to product, equipment, vehicles or process not directly attributable to the accident (e.g. caused by replacement staff);
▶ increases in insurance premiums resulting from the accident;

▶ any compensation not covered by the insurance policy due to an excess agreed between the employer and the insurance company; and

▶ legal representation following any compensation claim.

Indirect costs

Costs which may not be directly attributable to the accident but may result from a series of accidents.

Insured indirect costs include:

▶ a cumulative business loss;

▶ product or process liability claims; and

▶ recruitment of replacement staff.

Uninsured indirect costs include:

▶ loss of goodwill and a poor corporate image;

▶ accident investigation time and any subsequent remedial action required;

▶ production delays;

▶ extra overtime payments;

▶ lost time for other employees, such as a First-aider, who attend to the needs of the injured person;

▶ the recruitment and training of replacement staff;

▶ additional administration time incurred;

▶ first-aid provision and training; and

▶ lower employee morale, possibly leading to reduced productivity.

Some of these items, such as business loss, may be uninsurable or too prohibitively expensive to insure. Therefore, insurance policies can never cover all of the costs of an accident or disease, because either some items are not covered by the policy or the insurance excess is greater than the particular item cost.

Employers' liability compulsory insurance

▶ legal requirement for all employers;

▶ covers the employer's liability in the event of accidents and work-related ill-health to employees and others who may be affected by the operations;

7

► ensures that any employee who successfully sues his/her employer following an accident is assured of receiving compensation irrespective of the financial position of the employer; and

► made available either by display or electronically at each place of business.

Legal framework for health and safety

Sub-divisions of Law	
Criminal Law	**Civil Law**
► enforced by the State to punish individuals (and/or organisations)	► disputes between individuals (and/or organisations) to address a civil wrong (tort)
► individual is prosecuted by an Agency of the State (e.g. Police, HSE, Local Authorities, Fire Authority)	► individual(s) and/or organisations are sued
► individual(s) guilty or not guilty	► individual(s) are liable or not liable
► courts can impose fine or imprisonment	► courts can award compensation and costs
► proof 'beyond reasonable doubt'	► proof based on 'balance of probabilities'
► cannot insure against punishment	► employers must insure against civil actions (**Employers' Liability Insurance**)
Sources of Law	
Common Law	**Statute Law**
► based on judgments made by judges in courts	► law laid down by Acts of Parliament
► generally courts bound by earlier judgments (precedents)	► Health and Safety at Work Act 1974
► lower courts follow judgments of higher courts	► specific duties mainly in Regulations or Statutory Instruments
► in health and safety definitions of negligence, duties of care and terms such as 'practicable' and 'reasonably practicable' are based on common law judgments	► takes precedence over Common Law

Sub-divisions and sources of law

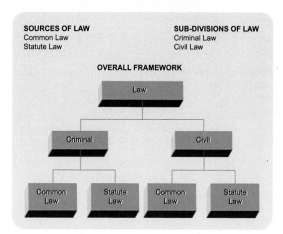

Figure 1 shows the relationship between the sub-divisions and sources of law

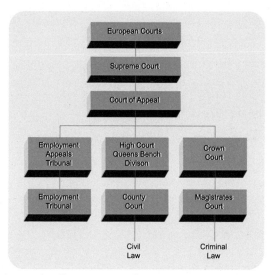

Figure 2 shows the Court system for health and safety in England and Wales

(NB European courts advise the Supreme Court)

Aspects of criminal law

The main prosecuting authorities in the UK are:

▶ the Crown Prosecution Service (CPS) in England and Wales;
▶ the Procurator Fiscal in Scotland; and
▶ the Public Prosecution Service for Northern Ireland (PPSNI) in Northern Ireland.

There are two types of criminal offence:

▶ Summary – minor offences, tried without a jury only in a magistrates court (or sheriff court in Scotland); and
▶ Indictable – most serious offences are called indictable offences and are tried only by the Crown Court (or the High Court of Justiciary in Scotland).

Comparison between English and Scottish courts

	Lower court	Higher court*
England and Wales	Magistrates	Crown
Scotland	Sheriff	High Court of Justiciary
Cases	Summary	Indictable

* Higher court deals with some summary cases referred to it by the lower court.

Aspects of civil law

Employer's common law duty of care

The employer has a duty of care to each for its employees. This duty cannot be assigned to another person. The duty of care falls into five categories, and the employer must provide:

▶ a safe place of work, including access and egress;
▶ a safe plant and equipment;
▶ a safe system of work;
▶ safe and competent fellow employees; and
▶ adequate levels of supervision, information, instruction and training.

Employees have a right not to be harmed in any way by their work, and they are expected to take reasonable care in their workplace.

Negligence

▶ lack of reasonable care or conduct resulting in injury, damage or loss
▶ it must be reasonably foreseeable that the acts or omissions could result in injury.

Defences against negligence claims	Partial defences against negligence claims
▶ a duty of care was not owed	▶ contributory negligence – employee contributed to the negligent act
▶ there was no breach of the duty of care	▶ volenti non fit injuria – the risk was willingly accepted by the employee
▶ any breach of a duty of care did not result in the specific injury, disease, damage and/or loss suffered	▶ acts of God, riot, terrorist event etc. ▶ a disagreement on the facts of the case

Negligence claims must be made within a set time.

Vicarious liability

When the defendant is acting in the normal course of his/her employment during the alleged incident, the defence of the action is transferred to the employer.

Tort of breach of statutory duty

This tort allows a person to seek compensation using a civil action following an accident or illness that resulted from a breach of statutory duty.

However, breaches of statutory duty, as described by regulations made under the HSW Act, only give rise to civil liability in cases concerning pregnant women or new mothers.

These employees may sue their employer both for negligence and for the breach of a statutory duty. Such an action is termed a **double-barrelled action**.

Levels of statutory duty

Absolute	Practicable	Reasonably practicable
The employer MUST comply with the law. Regulations use the verbs 'must' or 'shall'.	The employer must comply if it is technically possible. Difficulty, inconvenience or cost cannot be taken into account.	If the risk is small compared with the cost, time and effort required to further reduce the risk, then no action is required.

The legal framework for the regulation of health and safety

Influence of the European Union (EU)

▶ Role is to harmonise health and safety standards across member states
▶ Powers of EU in health and safety mainly derived from the Treaty of Rome (1957) and the Single European Act (1986)
▶ Article 95A (was 100A) – health and safety standards for plant and equipment
▶ Article 138A (was 118A) – minimum health and safety standards in employment
▶ European Directives set out the specific minimum aims of a given area of health and safety
▶ European Directives must be incorporated into the national law of all member states
▶ First introduction into UK law was in 1992 with the 'European Six Pack'
▶ European Court of Justice rules on interpretation of EU law
▶ European Court of Human Rights (covers a wider area than just the EU) interprets the European Human Rights Convention.

Health and safety at work act 1974

Background topics

The Health and Safety at Work Act (HSW Act) was introduced in 1974 and is a criminal law based on the recommendations of the Robens Report.

Main recommendations of the Robens Report

1 A single Act to cover all workers containing general duties
2 The Act should cover everyone affected by the employer's undertaking
3 Emphasis on management of health and safety, including training and supervision
4 Encouragement of employee involvement in accident prevention
5 Enforcement should be targeted at 'self-regulation' rather than prosecution.

The HSW Act is an **Enabling Act**, allowing regulations to be produced by the HSE on behalf of the Secretary of State without further Acts of Parliament being required.

The HSW Act contains mainly general duties, with specific duties defined in regulations.

Role and activities of the HSE

- ▶ advises on the development of regulations
- ▶ enforces health and safety regulations
- ▶ provides information to organisations (ACOPs, guidance notes, leaflets and other publications, accident and ill-health statistics)
- ▶ launches national health and safety campaigns on specific topics
- ▶ undertakes accident and other investigations
- ▶ offers advice to employers and others on statutory duties
- ▶ takes enforcement action
- ▶ instigates criminal proceedings and publicises organisations that receive enforcement notices.

Regulations

- ▶ state the law
- ▶ often implement EU Directives
- ▶ breaches are criminal offences possibly leading to enforcement action

- ▶ describe the minimum health and safety standards that need to be achieved
- ▶ usually apply across all organisations but sometimes apply to specific industries.

Approved Codes of Practice (ACOPs)

- ▶ supplementary practical interpretation of regulations that gives more detail on the regulatory requirements
- ▶ special legal status – quasi-legal because it may be possible to comply with regulations by some other more effective practice
- ▶ ACOPs are legally binding if the particular regulations indicate that they are or if they are quoted in an Enforcement Notice.

Guidance

- ▶ two forms of guidance – legal and best practice, both available as HSE publications
- ▶ not legally binding
- ▶ gives more informative and practical advice than ACOPs
- ▶ also often available as British Standards and as industrial or trade guidance.

The Health and Safety at Work Act

Section 2 duties of employers to employees

General duty – ensure, as far as is reasonably practicable, the health, safety and welfare of all employees.

Specific duties –

- ▶ safe plant and systems of work;
- ▶ safe use, handling, transport and storage of substances and articles;
- ▶ provision of information, instruction, training and supervision;
- ▶ safe place of work, access and egress;
- ▶ safe working environment with adequate welfare facilities;

- a written safety policy together with organisational and other arrangements (if five or more employees); and
- consultation with safety representatives and formation of safety committees where there are recognised trade unions.

Section 3 duties of employers to others affected by their undertaking

- 'others' could include contractors, general public, visitors, patients and students.

Section 4 duties of landlords or owners

- safe access and egress for those using the premises; and
- buildings and any equipment supplied with them are safe.

Section 6 duties of suppliers

Suppliers (including designers) of articles and substances for use at work to ensure, as far as is reasonably practicable, that

- articles are designed and constructed to be safe and without risk to health at all times when they are being set, cleaned, used and maintained;
- substances are similarly safe and without risk to health when being used, handled, stored or transported;
- arrange, where necessary, for suitable testing and examination; and
- supply suitable safety information and any revisions to customers.

Section 7 duties of employees

- take care for the health and safety of themselves and others who may be affected by their acts or omissions; and
- co-operate with their employer, as far as is necessary, to ensure compliance with any statutory health and safety duty.

Section 8

No person to misuse anything provided for health, safety or welfare purposes.

Section 9

Employees cannot be charged for health and safety requirements.

Enforcement of the Act

Fee for Intervention (FFI)

The Fee for Intervention (FFI) scheme places a duty on HSE to recover its costs for carrying out its regulatory functions from those found to be in **material breach** of health and safety law.

Written notification by an inspector of a material breach includes the following information:

▶ the law that the inspector's opinion relates to;
▶ the reasons for the opinion; and
▶ notification that a fee is payable to HSE.

Powers of inspectors

▶ enter premises at any reasonable time, accompanied by a police officer, if necessary;
▶ examine, investigate and require the premises to be left undisturbed;
▶ access to all records and other relevant documents;
▶ take samples and photographs, and, if necessary, dismantle and remove equipment or substances;
▶ seize, destroy or render harmless any substance or article;
▶ take statements;
▶ issue improvement and prohibition notices and, possibly, a formal caution; and
▶ initiate prosecutions.

Enforcement notices

Improvement notice

Issued for a specific breach of the law.

Appeal within 21 days to an Employment Tribunal – notice suspended until appeal is heard or withdrawn.

Prohibition notice

Issued to halt an activity that could lead to serious injury.

Appeal within 21 days to an Employment Tribunal – notice is not suspended.

Deferred prohibition notice – stops the work activity within a specified time limit.

Penalties	
Summary offences	**Indictable offences**
▶ for most health and safety offences up to £20,000 fine and/or up to 12 months' imprisonment	▶ unlimited fines for all health and safety offences
▶ up to five years' disqualification for convicted directors	▶ up to two years' imprisonment for all health and safety offences
	▶ up to 15 years' disqualification for convicted directors

The sentencing option of 12 months applies in Scotland but only applies in England and Wales when Section 154(1) of the Criminal Justice Act 2003 is enacted.

Work-related deaths

▶ Investigated by police initially to ascertain whether a charge of manslaughter (culpable homicide in Scotland) or corporate manslaughter is appropriate.

▶ If there are no such charges, the HSE or Local Authority continues the investigation.

17

The Corporate Manslaughter and Corporate Homicide Act

An organisation will have committed the new offence if:

▶ it owes a duty of care to another person in defined circumstances;

▶ there is a management failure by its senior managers; and

▶ it is judged that its actions or inaction amount to a gross breach of that duty resulting in a person's death.

The health and safety duties relevant to the Act are:

▶ employer and occupier duties including the provision of safe systems of work and training on any equipment used; and

▶ duties connected with

▷ the supply of goods and services to customers;

▷ the operation of any activity on a commercial basis;

▷ any construction and maintenance work; and

▷ the use or storage of plant, vehicles or any other item.

A breach of duty is gross if the organisation's management of health and safety falls far below that which would reasonably be expected.

On conviction, the offence is punishable by an unlimited fine, and the courts will be able to make:

▶ a remedial order requiring the organisation to take steps to remedy the management failure concerned;

▶ a publicity order requiring the organisation to publicise details of its conviction and fine; and

▶ an order to pay the costs of the prosecution and possibly compensation for bereavement and funeral expenses.

The publicity order requires an organisation convicted of corporate manslaughter to publicise:

▶ the fact that it has been convicted;

▶ the particulars of the offence;

▶ the amount of any fine; and

▶ the terms of any remedial order.

Employer duties and responsibilities

Under the HSW Act, the employer has a duty to safeguard the health, safety and welfare at work of:

▶ employees;
▶ other workers – agency, temporary or casual;
▶ trainees;
▶ contractors;
▶ visitors; and
▶ neighbours and the general public.

Key actions required of the employer

▶ ensure the availability of competent advice on health and safety matters;
▶ obtain current Employers' Liability insurance and display the certificate;
▶ compile a health and safety policy and ensure that an adequate health and safety management system is in place;
▶ ensure that risk assessments of all work activities are undertaken and any required controls are put in place;
▶ provide the workforce with health and safety information and training;
▶ provide adequate welfare facilities;
▶ consult the workforce on health and safety issues;
▶ report and investigate some accidents, diseases and dangerous occurrences; and
▶ display prominently the health and safety law poster (or supply workers with the appropriate leaflet).

The Working Time Regulations set a working limit averaging 48 hours a week (over a 17-week rolling reference period). Young workers must not work more than eight hours per day and 40 hours per week. Night workers are limited to an average of eight hours' work in a 24-hour period.

Other employer responsibilities

Visitors and the general public

Possible hazards	Possible controls
▶ unfamiliarity with the workplace processes	▶ visitor identification (use of badges)
▶ lack of knowledge of site layout	▶ routine signing in and out
▶ unfamiliarity with emergency procedures	▶ escorted by a member of staff
▶ inappropriate personal protective equipment	▶ provision of information on hazards and emergency procedures
▶ inadequate or unsigned walkways	▶ given explicit site rules (wearing of PPE)
▶ added vulnerability if young or disabled visitors	▶ clear marking of walkways

For night workers, employers should:

▶ determine the normal working time for night workers;

▶ if the working time is more than eight hours per day on average, determine whether the amount of hours can be reduced;

▶ develop an appropriate health assessment and method of making health checks;

▶ ensure that proper records of night workers are maintained, including details of health assessments; and

▶ ensure that night workers are not involved in work which is particularly hazardous.

Duties of managers and supervisors

Managers should:

▶ familiarise themselves with the health and safety management system of the organisation;

▶ ensure that there is an adequate and appropriate level of supervision for all workers;

▶ ensure that supervisors are aware of

  ▷ the health and safety standards of the organisation,

  ▷ the specific hazards within their area of supervision,

  ▷ the need to set a good example on health and safety issues,

▷ the need to monitor the health and safety performance of their workforce, and

▷ the training needs, including induction training, of their workforce;

▶ ensure that sufficient resources are available to allow tasks to be completed safely and without risks to health; and

▶ communicate to the Chief Executive and the Board the adherence or otherwise of the health and safety standards agreed by the Board.

Supervisors should lead by example in health and safety matters (such as the wearing of PPE) and ensure that:

▶ workers in their department understand the risks associated with their workplace and the measures available to control them;

▶ the risk control measures are up to date and are being properly used, maintained and monitored;

▶ particular attention is paid to new, inexperienced or young people and those whose first language is not English;

▶ workers are encouraged to raise concerns over any shortcomings in health and safety provision; and

▶ arrangements are in place to supervise the work of contractors.

Duties and responsibilities of employees and others

Employees and agency workers

Under the HSW Act, employees and agency workers have specific duties:

▶ take care for the health and safety of themselves and others who may be affected by their acts or omissions;

▶ co-operate with their employer, as far as is necessary, to ensure compliance with any statutory health and safety duty; and

▶ not to interfere with or deliberately misuse anything provided, in accordance with health and safety legislation, to further health and safety at work.

Self-employed

Under the HSW Act, the self-employed are:

▶ responsible for their own health and safety; and
▶ responsible for ensuring that others who may be affected by their undertaking are not exposed to risks to their health and safety.

In 2015, self-employed persons are exempted from the general duty in the HSW Act in respect of themselves and other persons (not being their employees), except those undertaking activities on a prescribed list defined by one of the following four criteria:

▶ there are high numbers of self-employed in a particular industry and high rates of injuries and/or fatalities (e.g. agriculture);
▶ there is a significant risk to members of the public (e.g. fairgrounds);
▶ there is the potential for mass fatalities (e.g. explosives); or
▶ there is a European obligation to retain the general duty on self-employed persons (e.g. construction – Council Directive 92/57/EEC imposes duties on the self-employed for safety and health requirements at temporary or mobile construction sites).

The occupational sectors for which no exemption is proposed include agricultural activities; construction; quarries; mining; diving; COMAH and sub-COMAH sites; offshore activities; nuclear installations; explosives; and gas-fitting and installation.

Persons in control of premises

The duty of 'Persons in control of **non-domestic** premises' under Section 4 of the HSW extends to:

▶ people entering the premises to work
▶ people entering the premises to use machinery or equipment
▶ access to and exit from the premises
▶ corridors, stairs, lifts and storage areas.

Duties of manufacturers and others in the supply chain

Section 6 of the HSW Act (covered earlier) requires persons who design, manufacture, import or supply any article or substance for use at work to ensure, so far as is reasonably practicable, that it is safe and without risk to health, and employers should be provided with information on the safe use, dismantling and disposal of the articles and substances and given revised information should a subsequent serious risk become known.

Importers have a duty to ensure articles or substances comply with the requirements of UK legislation.

Advantages of good supply chain management

▶ reduction of waste of materials and time;
▶ ability to respond rapidly to changing requirements at short notice;
▶ reduction in accidents due to close liaison;
▶ legal duties addressed satisfactorily; and
▶ easier to maintain good customer care.

Role and functions of external agencies

Office of Rail Regulation (ORR)

▶ responsible for the independent health and safety regulation of the railway industry in the UK;
▶ inspectors known as Her Majesty's Railway Inspectors.

Fire and rescue authority

▶ enforces fire safety law;
▶ undertakes random fire inspections (often to examine fire risk assessments);
▶ can issue alteration, improvement and prohibition notices; and
▶ needs to be informed during the planning stage of building alterations when fire safety of the building may be affected.

Environment agency (Scottish Environmental Agency)

▶ responsible for authorising and regulating emissions from industry;

▶ ensuring effective controls of the most polluting industries;

▶ monitoring radioactive releases from nuclear sites;

▶ ensuring that discharges to controlled waters are at acceptable levels;

▶ setting standards and issuing permits for the collection, transporting, processing and disposal of waste (including radioactive waste);

▶ enforcement of the Producer Responsibility Obligations (Packaging Waste) Regulations 1997; and

▶ enforcement of the Waste Electrical and Electronic Equipment (WEEE) Directive and its associated directives.

Insurance companies

▶ legal requirement for employers to insure against liability for injury or disease to their employees arising out of their employment;

▶ offer fire and public liability insurance; and

▶ can influence health and safety standards by weighting the premium offered to an organisation against its health and safety record.

Management of health and safety at work regulations

Employers' duties

▶ undertake suitable and sufficient written risk assessments (five or more employees);

▶ put in place effective health and safety management arrangements and record them if five or more employees;

▶ undertake preventative and protective measures on the basis of the principles of prevention specified in Schedule 1 to the regulations;

▶ employ a competent health and safety person;

▶ develop suitable emergency arrangements and inform employees and others;

▶ provide health and safety information to employees and others, such as other employers, the self-employed and their employees who are sharing the same workplace, and parents of child employees or those on work experience;

▶ co-operate in health and safety matters with other employers who share the same workplace;

▶ provide employees with adequate and relevant health and safety training;

▶ provide temporary workers and their contract agency with appropriate health and safety information;

▶ protect new and expectant mothers and young persons from particular risks; and

▶ under certain circumstances, as outlined in Regulation 6, provide health surveillance for employees.

The information that should be supplied by employers under the Regulations is the following:

▶ risks identified by any risk assessments, including those notified to them by other employers sharing the same workplace;

▶ the preventative and protective measures that are in place; and

▶ the emergency arrangements and procedures and the names of those responsible for the implementation of the procedures.

Employees' duties

▶ use any equipment or substance in accordance with any training or instruction given by the employer;

▶ report to the employer any serious or imminent danger; and

▶ report any shortcomings in the employer's protective health and safety arrangements.

Self-employed duties

▶ carry out appropriate risk assessment;
▶ co-operate with other people who work in the premises and, where necessary, in the appointment of a health and safety co-ordinator; and
▶ provide comprehensible information to other people's employees working in their premises.

Joint occupation of premises

The Regulations specifically state that where two or more employers share a workplace – whether on a temporary or a permanent basis – each employer shall:

▶ co-operate with other employers;
▶ take reasonable steps to co-ordinate between other employers to comply with legal requirements; and
▶ take reasonable steps to inform other employers where there are risks to health and safety.

Responsibilities of clients and their contractors

Contractors are protected by the HSW Act (Section 3). Most contracted work is governed by a legally binding contract that should cover all parts of the work and the principles of cooperation, coordination and communication between organisations.

The following points should be considered when contractors are employed:

▶ Health and safety must be included in the contract specification.
▶ All significant hazards must be included in the contract specification.
▶ The contractor must be selected with safety in mind.
▶ Prior to the start of work, health and safety policies should be exchanged.

▶ The contractor must be given basic site and health and safety information, such as welfare and first-aid arrangements, significant hazards, safe storage of chemicals and the name of the contract supervisor.

▶ Where appropriate, the contractor should supply risk assessments and method statements.

▶ For construction work, the contractor should be aware of the position of buried/overhead services and the arrangements for the disposal of waste.

▶ The contractor should be monitored during the progress of the contract by the contract supervisor.

▶ The contract supervisor should check that the work has been completed safely at the end of the contract.

The management of construction activities (CDM 2015 regulations)

The duty holders and their main duties are:

▶ The **Client** has a major role and must ensure that
  ▷ all duty holders are competent;
  ▷ HSE informed of notifiable projects;
  ▷ pre-construction information is passed to relevant duty holders (designers and contractors);
  ▷ a Principal Designer is appointed and complies with their duties under the Regulations including the preparation of a health and safety file for the project;
  ▷ a Principal Contractor is appointed and complies with their duties under the Regulations including the preparation of a construction phase plan;
  ▷ the welfare requirements in schedule 2 of the Regulations are followed;
  ▷ health and safety arrangements are maintained and reviewed throughout the project; and
  ▷ adequate resources and sufficient time are available for the safe completion of the work.

▶ **Domestic clients** are a special case and do not have specific duties under CDM 2015. Unless there is a written agreement between the domestic client and the principal designer, the duties of the client must be carried out by the contractor or principal contractor where there is more than one. Where no appointment is made, the first designer and contractor appointed are deemed to be the principal one in each case.

▶ The **Designer** must:

  ▷ ensure that adequate health and safety provision is incorporated into the design;

  ▷ provide adequate information about any significant risks associated with the design; and

  ▷ co-ordinate their work with that of the other duty holders.

▶ The **Principal Designer** must ensure that:

  ▷ the project is carried out safely so far as is reasonably practicable;

  ▷ assistance is given to client for the provision of pre-construction information;

  ▷ health and safety risks are identified, eliminated, controlled or reduced;

  ▷ the cooperation of everyone working on the project;

  ▷ the preparation and revision as necessary of the health and safety file;

  ▷ the provision of pre-construction information to every designer and contractor; and

  ▷ liaison with the principal contractor for the duration of the project particularly over the preparation of the construction phase plan.

▶ The **Principal Contractor** must ensure that:

  ▷ the health and safety construction phase plan is developed and managed;

  ▷ the construction phase is properly planned, managed and monitored;

  ▷ only competent sub-contractors are employed and supplied with necessary health and safety information;

28

▷ necessary site health and safety rules are drawn up and suitable site induction is provided;

▷ access by unauthorised persons is controlled preventing unauthorised access to the site;

▷ there is liaison with the principal designer throughout the project particularly regarding information for the health and safety file and management of the construction phase plan;

▷ the health and safety file is appropriately updated, reviewed and revised to take account of changes;

▷ suitable welfare facilities are provided on site; and

▷ the project notification is displayed.

▶ The **Contractor** must:

▷ not undertake construction work on a project unless satisfied that the client is aware of the client's duties under CDM2015;

▷ plan, manage and monitor the way construction work is done to ensure it is safe so far as is reasonably practicable;

▷ where there is no principal contractor, ensure that a construction phase plan is drawn up prior to setting up the site;

▷ provide any employees, or persons under their control, any information and instruction to ensure the safety of the project;

▷ ensure that the welfare requirements in schedule 2 of the regulations are provided for employees and others under their control;

▷ comply with any directions given by the principal designer or principal contractor and any site rules; and

▷ consult with their workers.

Required documentation

1 **Pre-construction information** – needs to identify the hazards and risks associated with the design and construction work.

2 **Health and safety file** – is a record of health and safety information required by the subsequent users of the finished construction project.

3 **Construction health and safety plan** – defines the organisation and arrangements required to control the site risks and co-ordinate the construction work.

4 **Notifiable work notice** – issued to the HSE if the construction work is to last longer than 30 days and has more than 20 workers simultaneously or involves more than 500 person days of work.

The principles of assessing and managing contractors

Scale of contractor use

The use of contractors has increased over recent years. Reasons include:

▶ the need to supplement permanent staff particularly for specialist tasks, or to undertake non-routine activities;

▶ the demand for products or services is uncertain;

▶ when more flexibility is required;

▶ contractors usually supply their own tools and equipment associated with the contract;

▶ there are no permanent staff available to perform the work;

▶ the financial overheads and legal employment obligations are lower;

▶ most of the costs associated with increasing and reducing employee numbers as product demand varies do not relate to contractors; and

▶ permanent staff can concentrate on the core business of the organisation.

There are some disadvantages in the use of independent contractors, including:

▶ contractors/subcontractors may cost more than the equivalent daily rate for employing a worker;

▶ by relying on contractors, the skills of permanent staff are not developed;

▶ there is less control over contractors than permanently employed staff (this can be a significant problem if the contractor sub-contracts some of the work); and

▶ the control of the contractor and the quality of the work is crucially dependent on the terms of the contract.

Selection of contractors

Most contracted work is governed by a legally binding contract, and it is, therefore, very important that the contract covers all parts of the work – for example, competent workers, safe access when working at height, fire precautions and safe waste disposal.

The following issues should be considered:

▶ an adequate health and safety policy;

▶ competent supervision;

▶ the availability of competent health and safety advice;

▶ past accident record;

▶ ability to assess hazards and risks involved in the contract and implement appropriate control measures;

▶ examples of method statements;

▶ a competent, trained and experienced workforce; and

▶ good references from previous contracts.

Management and authorisation of contractors

It is important that contractors are made aware of:

▶ the health and safety procedures and rules of the organisation;

▶ the hazards on the site, particularly those associated with the project;

▶ any special equipment or personal protective equipment that they need to use;

▶ the emergency procedures and the sound of the alarm; and

▶ the safe disposal of waste.

Contractors and their employees, and sub-contractors and their employees, should not be allowed to commence work on any client's site without **authorisation** signed by the company contact. The contact will need to check as a minimum the following:

▶ the correct contractor for the work has been selected;
▶ the contractor has made appropriate arrangements for supervision of staff;
▶ the contractor has received and signed for a copy of the contractor's safety rules;
▶ the contractor is clear what is required, the limits of the work and any special precautions, including permits to work, that need to be taken; and
▶ the contractor's personnel are properly qualified for the work to be undertaken.

Copies of the authorisation document should be retained by all contractors and a copy kept on site.

Safety rules for contractors

Contractors' safety rules should contain as a minimum the following points:

▶ **Health and safety** – that the contractor operates to at least the minimum legal standard and conforms to accepted industry good practice;
▶ **Supervision** – that the contractors provides a good standard of supervision of their own employees;
▶ **Sub-contractors** – that they may not use sub-contractors without prior written agreement from the organisation; and
▶ **Authorisation** – that each employee must carry an authorisation card issued by the organisation at all times while on site.

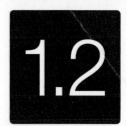

1.2

Health and safety management systems 1 – Plan

Learning outcomes

Outline the key elements of a health and safety management system	☐
Explain the purpose and importance of setting policy for health and safety	☐
Describe the key features and appropriate content of an effective health and safety policy	☐

🔑 **Key revision points**	
The four key elements of the health and safety management system HSG 65	☐
The legal requirements for a health and safety policy	☐
The three key elements of a health and safety policy	☐
Target setting for health and safety performance	☐
Circumstances leading to the need for a review of health and safety policy	☐
The reasons for unsuccessful health and safety policies	☐

Key elements of a health and safety management system (HSG 65)

The HSE document HSG65, Managing for health and safety, describes the occupational health and safety management system used extensively in the UK and is based on a 'Plan, Do, Check, Act' approach.

The four elements of HSG 65 are:

1 **PLAN** – the establishment of standards for health and safety management based on risk assessment and legal requirements and the formulation of a health and safety plan and policy.
2 **DO** – the implementation of the health and safety plan to achieve the policy objectives and standards. This will involve good communication, the promotion of competency, the commitment of all employees and a responsive reporting system.
3 **CHECK** – the measurement of progress with plans and compliance with standards and includes both active (sometimes called proactive) and reactive monitoring of the health and safety management system. It will measure the performance of the organisation against its own long-term goals and objectives and its progress with the health and safety plan and compliance with standards.

4 **ACT** – the review against objectives and standards and take appropriate action. The results of monitoring and independent audits are used to indicate whether the objectives and targets set in the health and safety policy need to be changed. Changes in the health and safety environment in the organisation, such as an accident, should also trigger a performance review.

The framework of health and safety management HSG 65

HSG 65 element	Main topics in each element	Components of each topic
PLAN	Health and safety policy Health and safety plan	Define health and safety aims, objectives and resources. Hazard identification and some risk assessment may be required. Plan should include emergency procedures (including first-aid), legal requirements and methods of performance measurement.
DO	Profile of health and safety risks Health and safety organisation Implementation of health and safety plan	Assess risks. Introduce and/or monitor risk controls. Designation of health and safety responsibilities. Ensure good communication, consultation, supervision and training of the workforce. Develop safe systems of work and, where appropriate, permit to work. Provide adequate resources, including competent advice where needed.
CHECK	Performance measurement Accident and incident investigation	Monitor the implementation of the health and safety plan using various inspection techniques. Investigate the causes of accidents, incidents or near misses and monitor any recommendations made.
ACT	Performance review Act on lessons learnt Continual improvement	Review health and safety performance using accidents and incidents, ill-health data and relative to benchmarks from similar organisations. Review plans, policy documents and risk assessments to see if they need updating. Take any required action following audit and inspection reports.

Planning a health and safety management system

The health and safety planning process begins with finding:

▶ the correct information about the existing management system for health and safety;

▶ suitable benchmarks against which to make comparisons; and

▶ competent people to carry out the analysis and make sensible judgements.

Further judgement may be necessary to establish if the system is:

▶ adequate for the organisation and the range of hazards/risks;

▶ working as intended and achieving the right objectives; and

▶ delivering cost-effective and proportionate risk control in the workplace.

Purpose and importance of setting policy for health and safety

The purpose of setting a health and safety policy is to ensure that:

▶ everybody associated with the organisation is aware of its health and safety aims and objectives and how they are to be achieved;

▶ the performance of the organisation is enhanced in areas other than health and safety;

▶ there is effective personal development of the workforce;

▶ business efficiency is improved throughout the operation; and

▶ the involvement of senior management in health and safety issues is evident to all stakeholders.

The policy should state the intentions of the business in terms of clear aims, objectives, organisation, arrangements and targets for all health and safety issues.

The law requires that the written health and safety policy should include the following three sections:

▶ a health and safety **policy statement of intent** which includes the health and safety aims and objectives of the organisation;

▶ the health and safety **organisation** detailing the people with specific health and safety responsibilities and their duties; and

▶ the health and safety **arrangements** in place in terms of systems and procedures.

Setting health and safety objectives

The standard of the health and safety objectives of an organisation will depend upon:

▶ the seniority of the person setting the objectives;

▶ the formal documentation associated with the objectives and their relevance at each functional level in the organisation;

▶ the prioritisation of targets to define the Key Performance Indicators (KPIs);

▶ the incorporation of relevant legal, technological options and good practice guidance;

▶ the identification and assessment of all significant hazards and risks within the organisation;

▶ the success with which they integrate with financial, operational and business requirements; and

▶ the incorporation of the views of employees, stakeholders and other interested parties.

The objectives must be **specific**, **measurable**, **achievable** and with **realistic timescales** (**SMART**) and kept up to date with any changes in legislation.

Legal requirements

Section 2 of the HSW Act and the Employers' Health and Safety Policy Statements (Exception) Regulations 1975 require employers with **five or more** employees to prepare and review on a regular basis a written health and safety policy, together with the necessary organisation and arrangements to carry it out and to bring the policy and any revision of it to the notice of their employees.

Policy statement of intent	Organisation	Arrangements to include
▶ Aims and objectives	▶ Safety manual	▶ Planning and organising
▶ Duties of employer and employees	▶ Organisational chart	▶ Accident reporting
▶ Performance targets and benchmarks	▶ Responsibilities	▶ Emergencies
▶ Name of person responsible for health and safety	▶ Allocation of resources including finance	▶ Contractors and visitors
▶ Posted and dated	▶ Safety monitoring system	▶ Consultation and communication with employees
	▶ Identification of main hazards	▶ Fire precautions
		▶ Main risk assessments and hazard control
		▶ Performance monitoring

Reasons for a review of the health and safety policy

▶ Significant organisational and/or technological changes have taken place.
▶ There have been changes in personnel and/or legislation.
▶ Health and safety performance has fallen below the occupational group's benchmarks.
▶ The monitoring of risk assessments and/or accident/incident investigations indicates that the health and safety policy is no longer totally effective.
▶ Enforcement action has been taken by the HSE or Local Authority.
▶ A sufficient period of time has elapsed since the previous review.

Benchmarking

Benchmarking compares the performance of the organisation with that of similar organisations. The advantages of benchmarking are that:

▶ the key performance indicators for a particular organisation may be easily identified;

▶ it helps with continuous improvement;
▶ it focuses attention on weaker performance areas;
▶ it gives confidence to various stakeholders; and
▶ it is useful feedback for boards, chief executives and managers.

The effects of a positive health and safety performance

are to:

▶ support the overall development of personnel;
▶ improve communication and consultation throughout the organisation;
▶ minimise financial losses due to accidents and ill-health and other incidents;
▶ directly involve senior managers in all levels of the organisation;
▶ improve supervision, particularly for young persons and those on occupational training courses;
▶ improve production processes; and
▶ improve the public image of the organisation or company.

The reasons for unsuccessful health and safety policies

include:

▶ the statements in the policy and the health and safety priorities are not understood by, or properly communicated to, the workforce;
▶ minimal resources are made available for the implementation of the policy;
▶ too much emphasis on rules for employees and too little on management policy;
▶ a lack of parity with other activities of the organisation (such as finance);
▶ lack of senior management involvement in health and safety;
▶ inadequate personal protective equipment;
▶ unsafe and poorly maintained machinery and equipment; and
▶ a lack of health and safety monitoring procedures.

Health and safety management systems 2 – Do 1

Outline the organisational health and safety roles and
responsibilities of employers, directors and managers ☐

Explain the concept of health and safety culture and its
significance in the management of health and safety in an
organisation ☐

Outline the human factors which influence behaviour at
work in a way that can affect health and safety ☐

Explain how health and safety behaviour at work can be
improved ☐

Key revision points

The health and safety roles and responsibilities of employers to their employees and others affected by their undertaking	☐
The health and safety roles and responsibilities of directors, managers and supervisors	☐
The competence and responsibilities of the health and safety practitioner/adviser	☐
The definition and importance of a health and safety culture	☐
The relationship between culture and performance	☐
The definition of human factors and their influence on the culture	☐
The development of a positive health and safety culture	☐
The importance of good communication	☐
The duties of employers to consult with the workforce	☐
The different forms of health and safety training	☐
The internal and external influences on the health and safety culture of an organisation	☐
The duties of employers to consult with the workforce	☐

Organisational health and safety roles and responsibilities of employers, directors and managers

Organisational health and safety responsibilities – employers

The organisational health and safety responsibilities of employers are closely linked to their statutory duties which are covered in detail in 1.1.

Organisational health and safety responsibilities – directors

Directors and Board members should ensure that:

▶ health and safety arrangements are properly resourced;
▶ competent health and safety advice is obtained;
▶ regular reports are received on health and safety performance;
▶ any new or amended health and safety legislation is implemented;
▶ risk assessments are undertaken;
▶ there are regular audits of health and safety management systems and risk control measures; and
▶ there is adequate consultation with employees on health and safety issues.

The four elements that boards need to incorporate into their management of health and safety are:

▶ planning the direction of health and safety;
▶ delivering the plan for health and safety;
▶ monitoring health and safety performance; and
▶ reviewing health and safety performance.

Effective health and safety performance comes from the top, and directors have both collective and individual responsibility for health and safety.

Directors and Board members must ensure that	Management of health and safety at Board level involves
▶ the health and safety of employees and others, such as members of the public, is protected; ▶ risk management includes health and safety risks and becomes a key business risk in board decisions; and ▶ health and safety duties imposed by legislation are followed.	▶ planning the direction of health and safety; ▶ delivering the plan for health and safety; ▶ monitoring health and safety performance; and ▶ reviewing health and safety performance.

Organisational health and safety responsibilities – managers

Managing directors / chief executives, line managers and supervisors play key roles in ensuring that the health and safety policy is delivered and monitored.

1 Managing Directors / Chief Executives

Managing Directors / Chief Executives are responsible for:

▶ the health and safety performance within the organisation;

▶ ensuring that adequate resources are available for the health and safety requirements within the organisation including the appointment of a senior member of the senior management with specific responsibility for health and safety;

▶ appointing one or more competent persons and adequate resources to provide assistance in meeting the organisation's health and safety obligations, including specialist help where appropriate;

▶ the establishment, implementation and maintenance of a health and safety programme for the organisation that encompasses all areas of significant health and safety risk;

▶ the approval, introduction and monitoring of all site health and safety policies, rules and procedures; and

▶ the review and possible revision annually of the effectiveness of the health and safety programme.

2 Departmental managers

The principal departmental managers may report to the Site Manager, Managing Director or Chief Executive. In particular, they:

▶ are responsible and accountable for the health and safety performance of their department;

▶ are responsible for the engagement and management of contractors and that they are properly supervised;

▶ must ensure that any machinery, equipment or vehicles used within the department are maintained, correctly guarded and meet agreed health and safety standards (copies of records of all maintenance, statutory and insurance inspections must be kept by the Departmental Manager);

▶ develop a training plan that includes specific job instructions for new or transferred employees and follow up on the training by supervisors (copies of records of all training must be kept by the Departmental Manager);

▶ personally investigate all lost workday cases and dangerous occurrences and report to their line manager. Progress any required corrective action.

3 Supervisors

The supervisors are responsible to and report to their Departmental Manager. In particular, they:

▶ are responsible and accountable for their team's health and safety performance;

▶ enforce all safe systems of work procedures that have been issued by the Departmental Manager;

▶ instruct employees in relevant health and safety rules, make records of this instruction and enforce all health and safety rules and procedures;

▶ supervise any contractors that are working within their area of supervision;

▶ enforce personal protective equipment requirements, check that it is being used and periodically appraise condition of equipment; and

▶ record any infringements of the personal protective equipment policy.

Health and safety adviser

The health and safety adviser must:

▶ be competent following the attainment of a health and safety qualification and training;

▶ report directly to senior management on matters of policy;

▶ keep up to date with technological advances and legislative changes;

▶ advise on the establishment of health and safety, maintenance and accident investigation procedures; and

▶ provide liaison with external agencies, such as the HSE, Fire Authorities, contractors, insurance companies and the public.

Concept of health and safety culture

The safety culture of an organisation is the product of individual and group values, attitudes, perceptions, competencies and patterns of behaviour that determine the commitment to, and the style and proficiency of, an organisation's health and safety management.

Features of a good health and safety culture

▶ leadership and commitment to health and safety throughout the organisation, which is demonstrated in a genuine and visible way;

▶ mutual trust throughout the organisation;

▶ acceptance that high standards of health and safety are achievable as part of a long-term strategy formulated by the organisation requiring sustained effort and interest;

▶ detailed risk assessments and control and monitoring procedures;

▶ a health and safety policy statement that conveys a sense of optimism and outlines short- and long-term health and safety objectives – such a policy should also include codes of practice and required health and safety standards;

▶ training, communication and consultation procedures to ensure ownership and participation in health and safety throughout the organisation;

▶ encouragement to the workforce to report potential hazards;

▶ health and safety systems for monitoring equipment, processes, behaviour and procedures and the prompt rectification of any defects; and

▶ prompt accident investigation and implementation of remedial actions.

Indicators of a health and safety culture

▶ accident/incident rates;
▶ accident frequency rate;
▶ sickness and absentee rates;
▶ resources available for health and safety;
▶ level of legal and other compliance;
▶ turnover rates for employees;
▶ level of complaints;
▶ selection and management of contractors;
▶ levels and effectiveness of communication and supervision;
▶ health and safety management structure; and
▶ level of insurance premiums.

Human factors

One in ten near misses = one accident.

90% accidents due to human error – 70% poor management.

Human factors are affected by the:

▶ Organisation
▶ Job
▶ Individual (personal) factors.

Organisation

▶ must have a positive health and safety culture;
▶ manage health and safety by providing leadership and involvement of senior managers;
▶ motivate the workforce to improve health and safety performance; and
▶ measure health and safety performance.

Job

▶ recognise possibility of human error;
▶ good ergonomics, equipment design and layout of workstation;
▶ clear job descriptions;

▶ safe systems of work and operating procedures;
▶ job rotation and regular breaks;
▶ provision of correct tools; and
▶ effective training schedule and good communication.

Individual (personal) factors

The three common psychological factors are:

▶ attitude – tendency to behave in a particular way in a given situation, influenced by social background and peer pressure;
▶ motivation – the driving force behind the way a person acts or is stimulated to act;
▶ perception – the way in which a person believes or understands information supplied or a situation.

Other related factors:

▶ self-interest – e.g. effect of bonus systems;
▶ position in the team;
▶ acknowledgement by management of good work/initiatives;
▶ hearing and/or memory loss;
▶ experience and competence;
▶ age, personality, attitude, language problems;
▶ training undertaken and information given;
▶ effect of shift working – e.g. night working; and
▶ health (physical and mental).

Language and communication issues may be particular problems for some migrant workers.

The following negative factors can also affect the individual:

▶ low skill and competence levels;
▶ tired colleagues;
▶ bored or disinterested colleagues;
▶ individual medical or mental problems;
▶ complacency from repetitive tasks and lack of awareness training;
▶ inexperience especially if the employee is new or a young person; and
▶ peer pressure to conform to the 'group' or an individual's perception of how a task should be completed.

Human errors may be:	Violations may be:
1 Slips – failure to carry out the correct actions of a task	**1** Routine – the breaking of a safety rule or procedure is the normal way of working
2 Lapses – failure to carry out particular actions that form part of a working procedure	**2** Situational – job pressures at a particular time make rule compliance difficult
3 Mistakes: ▶ rule-based – a rule or procedure is applied or remembered incorrectly or ▶ knowledge-based – well-tried methods or calculation rules are applied incorrectly	**3** Exceptional – a safety rule is broken to perform a new task

Methods of improving health and safety behaviour at work

Development of a positive health and safety culture

By:

1 Commitment of management is the most important factor:
  ▶ Proactive management
  ▶ Promotion by example (e.g. wearing PPE).
2 The promotion of health and safety standards for:
  ▶ Selection and design of premises
  ▶ Selection and design of plant, processes and substances
  ▶ Recruitment of employees and contractors
  ▶ Risk assessments and control implementation
  ▶ Competence, maintenance and supervision
  ▶ Emergency planning and training
  ▶ Transportation of the product and its subsequent maintenance and servicing.
3 Competence of the workforce, including in health and safety:
  ▶ Knowledge and understanding of the work/job
  ▶ Capacity to apply knowledge to the particular task
  ▶ Awareness of one's limitations.

Identifying and keeping up to date with legal requirements

The comparison with legal standards and requirements is an essential part of the setting of health and safety objectives and can be achieved by:

▶ Regular checking of the HSE web site;
▶ Free subscription to HSE bulletins on the internet;
▶ Reading various health and safety periodicals;
▶ Reading journals or web sites of trade associations; or
▶ Reading the text of legislation on-line.

Communication

▶ Verbal (by mouth) – conversations, telephone
▶ Written – memos, emails, meeting minutes, data sheets
▶ Graphic – safety signs, posters, charts.

Use of notice boards

The limitations of notice boards include:

▶ the information may not be read;
▶ the notice boards may not be accessible;
▶ the information may become out-dated or defaced;
▶ some employees may not be able to read while others may not understand what they have read;
▶ there may be language barriers;
▶ the information is mixed in with other non-health and safety information; and
▶ there is no opportunity offered for feedback.

Alternative methods of communication include:

▶ memos, emails and company intranet;
▶ tool box talks and team briefings;
▶ induction training and any further back up training sessions;
▶ newsletters, bulletins and payslips;
▶ digital video media including DVDs;
▶ a staff handbook; and
▶ through safety committees, safety representatives, and representatives of employee safety.

50

The approved poster entitled *Health and Safety Law – what you should know* must be displayed on a notice board or the approved leaflet distributed.

In addition to the health and safety poster, the following types of health and safety information could be displayed on a workplace notice board:

▶ a copy of the Employers' Liability Insurance Certificate;
▶ details of first-aid arrangements;
▶ emergency evacuation and fire procedures;
▶ minutes of the last health and safety committee meeting;
▶ details of health and safety targets and performance against them; and
▶ health and safety posters and campaign details.

Barriers to effective communication

▶ language and dialect
▶ acronyms and jargon
▶ various physical and mental disabilities
▶ attitudes and perception of workers and supervisors.

Types of accident propaganda

▶ Statistics
▶ Films, DVDs and posters
▶ Targets
▶ Records.

For safety propaganda to be effective, it must have:

▶ a simple understandable message
▶ a positive believable message
▶ an appealing format that will motivate the reader.

Consultation with employees

Difference between informing and consulting:

▶ 'informing' is a one-way process involving the provision of relevant information by management to workers; whereas

▶ 'consulting' is a two-way process where account is taken of the views of workers before any decision is taken.

The benefits of consultation include:

▶ an improved health and safety culture;
▶ motivation of staff;
▶ reduction in accidents and ill health; and
▶ improved overall performance of the organisation.

Safety representatives from a recognised trade union have the following rights:

▶ to investigate accidents and dangerous occurrences;
▶ to investigate health and safety complaints;
▶ to undertake workplace inspections;
▶ to receive information from health and safety inspectors;
▶ to attend health and safety committee meetings;
▶ to have access to suitable facilities to perform their functions; and
▶ to be allowed time off with pay for health and safety training.

If two or more representatives request in writing for a health and safety committee to be set up, then the employer must comply within three months.

Representatives of Employee Safety (ROES) were established under the Consultation with Employees Regulations.

The employer must **inform** and **consult** employees on health and safety matters.

Difference between informing and consulting:

▶ 'informing' is a one-way process involving the provision of relevant information by management to workers; whereas
▶ 'consulting' is a two-way process where account is taken of the views of workers before any decision is taken.

ROES have the following functions:

▶ inform the employer of health and safety concerns of the workforce;
▶ inform the employer of potential hazards and dangerous occurrences in the workplace;

▶ inform the employer of any general matters that affect the health and safety of the workforce; and

▶ speak on behalf of the workforce to health and safety inspectors.

Employer must consult on:

▶ new processes or equipment or any changes in them;

▶ the appointment arrangements for a health and safety competent person;

▶ the results of any risk assessments;

▶ the arrangements for the management of health and safety training; and

▶ the introduction of new technologies.

Types of information that employer does NOT need to disclose if it:

▶ violates a legal prohibition

▶ endangers national security

▶ relates to a specific individual

▶ could harm the company commercially

▶ was obtained from legal proceedings.

Safety committees

Terms of reference should include the following:

▶ the study of accident and notifiable disease statistics to enable reports to be made of recommended remedial actions;

▶ the examination of health and safety audits and statutory inspection reports;

▶ the consideration of reports from the external enforcement agency;

▶ the review of new legislation, Approved Codes of Practice and Guidance and their effect on the organisation;

▶ the monitoring and review of all health and safety training and instruction activities in the organisation;

▶ the monitoring and review of health and safety publicity and communication throughout the organisation;

▶ the development of safe systems of work and safety procedures;

53

▶ the reviewing risk assessments;

▶ the considering reports from safety representatives; and

▶ the continuous monitoring of arrangements for health and safety and revising them whenever necessary.

Types of health and safety training

▶ Induction – at recruitment

▶ Job-specific

▶ Supervisory and management

▶ Specialist (e.g. first-aid)

▶ Refresher or reinforcement.

Internal influences on health and safety culture	External influences on health and safety culture
Management commitment	Expectations of society
Production/service demands	Legislation and enforcement
Communication	Insurance companies
Competence	Trade unions
Employee representation	State of the economy
	Commercial stakeholders

Health and safety management systems 2 – Do 2

Learning outcomes

Explain the principles and practice of risk assessment	☐
Explain the general principles of control and a general hierarchy of risk reduction measures	☐
Identify the key sources of health and safety information	☐
Explain what factors should be considered when developing and implementing a safe system of work for general activities	☐
Explain the role and function of a permit-to-work system	☐
Outline the need for emergency procedures and the arrangements for contacting emergency services	☐
Outline the requirements for, and effective provision of, first-aid in the workplace	☐

Key revision points

The legal requirements for a health and safety risk assessment	☐
The meaning of 'suitable and sufficient'	☐
The forms and objectives of risk assessment	☐
Details of accident categories and types of health risks	☐
The risk assessment process and its management	☐
Groups that require a special risk assessment	☐
The principles of prevention and the hierarchy of risk control	☐
The development and application of safe systems of work and permits to work for various activities, including those in confined spaces	☐
Hazards and controls for confined spaces and machinery maintenance work	☐
The development of emergency and first-aid procedures in the workplace	☐

Principles and practice of risk assessment

Legal requirement

Regulation 3 of Management of Health and Safety at Work Regulations requires written suitable and sufficient risk assessment if there are five or more employees.

Suitable and sufficient means:

▶ identify significant risks only;
▶ identify measures required to comply with legislation; and
▶ remain appropriate and valid over a reasonable period of time.

Hazard – the potential to cause harm

Risk – the likelihood to cause harm

Residual risk – the risk remaining after some controls are in place.

Forms of risk assessment

▶ Quantitative – calculated from risk = likelihood × severity
▶ Qualitative – descriptor (high, medium or low) used to describe timetable for remedial action
▶ Generic – covers similar activities or work equipment.

Health risks

▶ Chemical – exhaust fumes, paint solvents, asbestos
▶ Biological – legionella, pathogens, hepatitis
▶ Physical – noise, vibration, radiation
▶ Psychological – stress, violence
▶ Ergonomic – musculoskeletal disorders.

Risk assessment team requirements

▶ all need training in risk assessment
▶ leader should have health and safety experience
▶ all need to be competent to assess risks in area under examination
▶ all need to know their own limitations
▶ include local line manager in the team
▶ at least one team member with report writing skills.

Risk assessment process

▶ **Hazard identification – Step 1** of HSE's five steps
▶ **Persons at risk – Step 2** of HSE's five steps
　▷ employees, agency/temporary workers, contractors, shift workers
　▷ members of the public – visitors, customers, patients, students, children, elderly
　▷ special groups – young persons, expectant or nursing mothers, workers with a disability, lone workers.

57

► **Evaluation of risk level (residual risk) – Step 3** of HSE's five steps
  ▷ high, medium and low (defined qualitatively or quantitatively)
  ▷ both occupational and organisational risk levels need to be considered.
► **Detail risk controls (existing and additional) – Step 3** of HSE's five steps
  ▷ the prioritisation of risk control is important
  ▷ risks can be reduced at the design stage by using the principles of prevention
  ▷ risks can be controlled by using the hierarchy of risk control.

Hierarchy of risk control

The health and safety management system ISO 45001 hierarchy of risk control is:

(a) eliminate the hazard;

(b) substitute with less hazardous materials, processes, operations or equipment;

(c) use engineering controls;

(d) use safety signs, markings and warning devices and administrative controls;

(e) use personal protective equipment.

There are several other similar hierarchies of risk control, which have been used over many years. A typical example is as follows:

1 elimination
2 substitution
3 changing work methods/patterns
4 reduced time exposure
5 engineering controls (isolation, insulation and ventilation)
6 good housekeeping
7 safe systems of work
8 training and information
9 personal protective equipment
10 welfare
11 monitoring and supervision
12 review.

Safety signs

 ▷ Red – prohibition – round (e.g. no smoking)
 ▷ Yellow – warning – triangular (e.g. wet floor)
 ▷ Blue – mandatory – round (e.g. ear defenders must be worn)
 ▷ Green – safe condition – square or rectangular (e.g. first aid).

▶ **Record of risk assessment findings – Step 4** of HSE's five steps

▶ **Monitor and review – Step 5** of HSE's five steps

Regular reviews required but need to be more frequent if:

 ▷ new legislation introduced
 ▷ new information available on substances or process
 ▷ changes to the workforce – introduction of trainees
 ▷ an accident has occurred.

Special cases

1 Young persons

▶ are under 18 years
▶ covered by Regulation 19 MHSWR
▶ subject to peer pressure and are inexperienced
▶ are eager to please
▶ appropriate level and approach of subject matter in training sessions.

There are additional requirements if under school leaving age.

A special risk assessment must be made to include details of:

▶ the work activity;
▶ any prohibited processes or equipment;
▶ the health and safety training provided; and
▶ the supervision arrangements.

2 Expectant and nursing mothers

There are restrictions on the type of work that can be undertaken.

Risks include:

▶ manual handling;
▶ chemical and biological agents;

- ionising radiation;
- passive smoking;
- lack of rest room facilities;
- temperature variations;
- prolonged standing or sitting;
- whole body vibration;
- issues associated with the use and wearing of personal protective equipment;
- working excessive hours;
- night working; and
- stress and violence to staff.

3 Workers with a disability

- emergency arrangements including 'raising the alarm'; and
- adequate wheelchair access to fire exit.

The special risk assessment should identify:

- the jobs with particular health and fitness requirements;
- the types of disability that would make certain jobs unsuitable; and
- the staff whose disabilities would exclude them from undertaking those jobs safely.

4 Lone workers

- special risk assessment (including violence);
- must be fit to work alone;
- special training should be given;
- possible to handle all equipment and substances alone;
- periodic visits by supervisor;
- regular mobile phone contact with base;
- first aid arrangements; and
- emergency arrangements.

General principles of control

The planning and implementing section of the health and safety management system is based on risk assessment and concerns all the actions taken to control or eliminate hazards and reduce risks. The principles of prevention are used when equipment or processes are being designed or selected. The hierarchy of risk control enables risk to be further controlled.

The principles of prevention

- ▶ avoid risks
- ▶ evaluate risks which cannot be avoided
- ▶ adapt work to the individual
- ▶ adapt to technical changes
- ▶ replace dangerous items with less dangerous items
- ▶ develop an overall prevention policy
- ▶ give priority to collective measures (Safe Place strategy)
- ▶ give instructions to employees (Safe Person strategy).

Sources of information on health and safety

Internal sources	External sources
▶ accident and ill-health records and investigation reports ▶ absentee records ▶ inspection and audit reports undertaken by the organisation and by external organisations such as the HSE ▶ maintenance, risk assessment (including COSHH) and training records	▶ health and safety legislation ▶ HSE publications, such as approved codes of practice, guidance documents, leaflets, journals, books and their website ▶ international (e.g. ILO), European and British standards ▶ health and safety magazines and journals
▶ documents which provide information to workers ▶ any equipment examination or test reports	▶ information published by trade associations, employer organisations and trade unions ▶ specialist technical and legal publications ▶ information and data from manufacturers and suppliers ▶ the internet and encyclopaedias

Development and implementation of safe systems of work

Employer's duty

This is contained in the common law duty of care and in Section 2 of the Health and Safety at Work Act.

Role of competent persons

A competent person or safety adviser should:

▶ assist managers to draw up guidelines for safe systems of work;
▶ prepare suitable documentation; and
▶ advise management on the adequacy of the safe systems produced.

Role of managers

▶ provide safe systems of work;
▶ ensure that employees are adequately trained in a specific safe system of work and are competent to carry out the work safely; and
▶ provide sufficient supervision to ensure that the system of work is followed and the work is carried out safely.

Employee involvement

Includes:

▶ consultation with those employees who will be exposed to the risks, either directly or through their representatives;
▶ discussion of the proposed system with those who will have to work under it and supervise it; and
▶ understanding that employees have a responsibility to follow the safe system of work.

Steps in the development of a safe system of work

1 Assess the task (complexity, accident records etc.)
2 Identify the significant hazards associated with the task
3 Define safe methods for performing the task (including emergency procedures) – document the methods if required
4 Implement the safe system of work (written safe system to be signed off)
5 Monitor the safe system of work and review it if necessary
6 Train the workforce in safe procedures and enter on training record.

Safe systems of work are particularly important for:

▶ maintenance work
▶ contractors
▶ emergency procedures
▶ lone working
▶ vehicle operations
▶ cleaning operations.

Method statements are formal written safe systems of work and are often used in construction work.

The safe system of work should be based on a thorough analysis of the job or operation to be covered by the system. After the introduction of a safe system of work the following controls are required:

▶ Engineering or process controls (e.g. guarding)
▶ Documented procedures
▶ Behavioural controls requiring a certain standard of behaviour from individuals.

Procedures for lone workers may include:

▶ periodic visits from the supervisor;
▶ regular voice contact;

▶ automatic warning devices to alert others of problems;
▶ checks that the lone worker has returned safely;
▶ special arrangements for first aid to deal with minor injuries; and
▶ emergency arrangements.

Specific examples of safe systems of work

Confined spaces

A confined space is defined in **Confined Spaces Regulations** as:

any place, including any chamber, tank, vat, silo, pit, trench, pipe, sewer, flue, well or other similar space in which, by virtue of its enclosed nature, there arises a reasonably foreseeable specified risk.

The principal hazards associated with a confined space include:

▶ difficult access and egress;
▶ asphyxiation due to oxygen depletion;
▶ poisoning by toxic substance or fumes;
▶ explosions due to gases, vapours and dust;
▶ fire due to flammable liquids;
▶ fall of materials leading to possible head injuries;
▶ free flowing solid such as grain in a silo;
▶ electrocution from unsuitable equipment;
▶ difficulties of rescuing injured personnel;
▶ drowning due to flooding; and
▶ fumes from plant or processes entering confined spaces.

The following topics need to be addressed in a safe system of work for a confined space:

▶ the appointment of a supervisor;
▶ the competence and experience required of the workers in the confined space;
▶ the isolation of mechanical and electrical equipment in an emergency;
▶ the size of the entrance must enable rapid access and exit in an emergency;

- the provision of adequate ventilation;
- the testing of the air inside the space to ensure that it is fit to breathe – if the air inside the space is not fit to breathe, then breathing apparatus will be essential;
- the provision of special tools and lighting, such as extra low voltage equipment, non-sparking tools and specially protected lighting;
- the emergency arrangements to cover the necessary equipment, training, practice drills and the raising of the alarm; and
- adequate communications arrangements to enable communication between people inside and outside the confined space and to summon help in an emergency.

Lone working

Typical control procedures may include:

- documented records of the location or itineraries of the lone workers;
- periodic visits from the supervisor to observe what is happening;
- regular voice contact, using mobile phones or radios, between the lone worker and the supervisor;
- automatic warning devices to alert others if a specific signal is not received from the lone worker;
- other devices to raise the alarm, which are activated by the absence of some specific action;
- checks that the lone worker has returned safely home or to their base;
- special arrangements for first-aid to deal with minor injuries – this may include mobile first-aid kits;
- arrangements for emergencies – these should be established and employees trained.

Role and function of a permit-to-work

Permits to work are:

- **formal** safe systems of work;
- required to be signed on/off by a responsible person; and

▶ often require equipment to be locked on/off by a responsible person.

To be used whenever there is a high risk of serious injury, such as:

▶ confined spaces
▶ live electricity (particularly high voltage)
▶ hot working (e.g. welding work)
▶ some machinery maintenance work.

Typical responsible persons are:

▶ site manager
▶ senior authorised person – often the chief engineer
▶ authorised person – issues permit
▶ competent person – receives permit
▶ operatives – supervised by a competent person
▶ specialists (e.g. electrical engineer)
▶ engineers – usually responsible for the work
▶ contractors.

The permit document should specify the following key items of information:

▶ the date, time and duration of the permit;
▶ a description and assessment of the task to be performed and its location;
▶ the plant/equipment involved, and how it is identified;
▶ the authorised persons to do the work;
▶ the steps which have already been taken to make the plant safe;
▶ potential hazards which remain, or which may arise as the work proceeds;
▶ the precautions to be taken against these hazards;
▶ the length of time that the permit is valid;
▶ the equipment to be released to those who are to carry out the work.

The permit will also include spaces for:

▶ signature certifying that the work is complete; and
▶ signature confirming re-acceptance of the plant/equipment.

Typical work tasks that might require a permit-to-work

Hot work

Typical controls include:

▶ a suitable fire extinguisher nearby;
▶ prompt removal of flammable waste material; and
▶ the damping down of nearby wooden structures such as floors.

Work on high-voltage apparatus (including testing)

Work on high-voltage apparatus (over about 600 V) is potentially high risk.

Hazards include:

▶ possible fatal electric shock/burns to the people doing the work;
▶ electrical fires/explosions;
▶ consequential danger from disruption of power supply to safety-critical plant and equipment.

Confined spaces

Examples include underground chamber, silo, trench, sewer and tunnel.

Hazards are:

▶ lack of oxygen and asphyxiation
▶ poor ventilation
▶ presence of fumes
▶ poor means of access and escape
▶ drowning
▶ claustrophobia
▶ electrical equipment (needs to be flameproof)
▶ presence of dust (e.g. silos)
▶ heat and high temperatures
▶ fire and/or explosion
▶ poor or artificial lighting.

Controls include:

▶ permit-to-work
▶ risk assessment
▶ training and information for all workers entering the confined space
▶ emergency arrangements in place
▶ emergency training
▶ no entry for unauthorised persons.

Machinery maintenance work

Hazards are:

▶ no perceived risk
▶ no safe system of work
▶ poor communications
▶ failure to brief contractors
▶ lack of familiarity
▶ poor design.

Control of hazards requires:

▶ effective planning
▶ a written safe system of work / permit-to-work
▶ a risk assessment to assess, control and reduce risks
▶ monitoring to ensure that the system of work and controls are used
▶ an effective training programme for all involved in the work.

Work at height

A permit-to-work may be required for some hazardous work at height, such as roof work, to ensure that a fall arrest strategy is in place. This is particularly important where:

▶ there are no permanent work platforms with fixed handrails on flat roofs;
▶ there are sloping or fragile roofs;
▶ specialist access equipment, like rope hung cradles, are required; and
▶ access is difficult.

68

Emergency procedures

Examples of types of emergencies

- ▶ fire
- ▶ explosions, bomb scares
- ▶ escape of toxic gases
- ▶ major accident.

Typical elements of emergency procedures

- ▶ Fire notices and fire procedures (including testing)
- ▶ Fire drills and evacuation procedures
- ▶ Assembly and roll call
- ▶ Arrangements for contacting emergency and rescue services
- ▶ Provision of information for emergency services
- ▶ Internal emergency organisation – including control of spillages and clean-up arrangements
- ▶ Media and publicity arrangements
- ▶ Business continuity arrangements.

Testing and training for emergencies

Training courses should be given to staff on a regular basis on the following topics:

- ▶ use of fire-fighting equipment;
- ▶ regular refresher first-aid training;
- ▶ suitable training (and competency assessment) for all those allocated particular roles in an emergency; and
- ▶ regular timed fire drills.

Provision of first-aid

Main functions of first-aid treatment

- ▶ preservation of life and/or minimisation of the consequences of serious injury until medical help is available
- ▶ treatment of minor injuries not needing medical attention.

Main first-aid requirements

▶ qualified first-aiders
▶ adequate facilities and equipment to administer first-aid
▶ an assessment of required first-aid cover and requirements
▶ an appointed person available to assist first-aiders.

Basic first-aid provision (including number of first-aiders)

Depends on:

▶ number of workers;
▶ the hazards and risks in the workplace;
▶ accident record and types of injuries;
▶ proximity to emergency medical services; and
▶ working patterns (shift work).

First-aider requires first-aid training, and the first-aid course depends on the level of risk in the workplace.

▶ For low risk, a six-hour Emergency First-aid at Work course
▶ For higher risk, 18-hour First-aid at Work course
▶ Either six-hour emergency or four-day first-aid course initially
▶ A repeat course every three years.

Appointed person has some other first-aid experience/ qualification.

First-aid box – contents depend on particular workplace needs but should be checked regularly.

Health and safety management systems 3 – Check

Key revision points

The reasons for measuring and monitoring health and safety performance	☐
The role of standards in the monitoring process	☐
The differences between reactive and active (proactive) monitoring	☐
The importance of clear, unambiguous report writing	☐
The reasons and legal requirements for recording and reporting incidents and accidents	☐
Basic accident investigation procedures and the different types of accident and incident	☐
Immediate and underlying causes of incidents	☐
Issues concerning insurance and compensation claims	☐

Active and reactive monitoring

Reactive monitoring (taking action after a problem occurs) involves	Proactive (or active) monitoring (taking action before problems occur) involves
▶ review of accident and ill-health reports – often to check that remedial advice has been actioned or ascertain trends and hot spots	▶ the active monitoring of the workplace for unsafe conditions
▶ review of procedures following dangerous occurrences, other property damage and near misses	▶ the direct observation of workers for unsafe acts
▶ review of compensation claims	▶ meeting with management and workers to discover any problems
▶ review of complaints from the workforce and members of the public	▶ checking documents, such as maintenance records, near miss reports, insurance reports
▶ review of procedures following enforcement reports and notices	▶ undertaking workplace inspections, sampling, surveys, tours and audits
▶ review of risk assessments following the discovery of additional hazards	

Workplace inspections

Detailed check, often using a checklist, of the whole workplace and should cover:

▶ the premises (e.g. fire precautions, access/egress, housekeeping);
▶ the plant, equipment and substances (e.g. machine guarding, tools, ventilation);
▶ the procedures in place (e.g. safe systems of work, risk assessments, use of PPE); and
▶ the workforce (e.g. training, information, supervision, health surveillance).

Other issues with inspections

▶ the competence of the observers;
▶ the frequency of inspections;
▶ the response to the inspection report; and
▶ the use of objective inspection standards.

Safety sampling – checking for safety defects in a selected area of the workplace (e.g. all fire extinguishers).

Safety surveys – a detailed inspection of a particular workplace activity throughout an organisation (e.g. manual handling).

Safety tours – an unscheduled brief inspection of a work area in the workplace by a team led by a senior manager.

Investigating incidents

Purpose of accident/incident investigation is to:

▶ eliminate the cause and future occurrences;
▶ determine the direct and indirect causes of the accident/incident;
▶ define any corrective and/or preventative actions;
▶ identify any deficiencies in risk controls, the health and safety management system and/or procedures;
▶ ensure that all legal requirements are being met; and
▶ comply with the recommendations of the Woolf Report so that essential information is available in the event of a civil claim.

Benefits of accident/incident investigation:

▶ prevention of a recurrence;

▶ prevention of future business losses;

▶ prevention of future increased insurance premiums and costs of criminal and civil actions; and

▶ improve employee morale and organisation reputation.

Accident triangles and their limitation

Accident triangles indicate the ratio between fatalities, serious accidents and minor accidents (sometimes near misses are included). The limitations of these triangles are:

▶ similar injuries may have different causes;

▶ some incidents have the potential for serious injury yet may only result in a minor one;

▶ serious injuries have different underlying causes to minor injuries; and

▶ many injuries are musculoskeletal sprains and strains which do not result in fatal injuries.

Accident causation

Direct or immediate include	Indirect, root or underlying include
▶ unsafe acts by individuals due to poor behaviour or a lack of training, supervision, information or competence or a failure to wear PPE ▶ unsafe conditions, such as inadequate guarding, inadequate procedures, hazardous substances, ergonomic and/or environmental factors ▶ fire or explosive hazards	▶ poor machine maintenance and/or start-up procedures ▶ management and social pressures ▶ financial restrictions ▶ lack of management commitment to health and safety ▶ poor or lack of health and safety policy and standards ▶ poor workplace health and safety culture ▶ workplace and trade customs and attitudes

Elements of an investigation

▶ interview relevant operatives, managers, supervisors
▶ obtain detailed plans and/or photographs of scene
▶ check all relevant records (working procedures, maintenance, training, risk assessments)
▶ interview all witnesses
▶ possibly arrange for equipment and/or substances to be independently tested
▶ produce a concise report for management that includes
  ▷ background to the accident
  ▷ possible causes of the accident (direct and indirect)
  ▷ relevant health and safety legislation, guidance and standards
  ▷ recommendations (including any remedial actions)
  ▷ any additional training or follow-up requirements
▶ undertake a post-accident risk assessment.

Recording and reporting incidents

Accident reporting requirements

▶ the organisational accident/incident report form
▶ accident book
▶ RIDDOR 2013 – records kept for three years.

RIDDOR 2013

The Regulations apply to employees, the self-employed, trainees and contractors. Any fatality or injury to a member of the public resulting in off-site medical treatment is reportable.

Fatality	▶ reportable by quickest means (telephone)
	▶ submit online form immediately
	▶ submit a report within ten days
	▶ reportable if death occurs within one year of accident

Specified serious injury/ ill-health	▶ reportable as soon as possible
	▶ submit online form immediately
	▶ submit a report within ten days
	▶ examples – any fracture, other than fingers, thumbs or toes; any amputation; any other injury requiring admittance to hospital for more than 24 hours
Over seven days' lost time injury	▶ submit online form within 15 days
Disease	▶ submit online form as soon as diagnosis is confirmed
	▶ examples – hepatitis; occupational dermatitis; hand-arm vibration syndrome
Dangerous occurrence	▶ a 'near miss' that could lead to serious injury or loss of life.
	▶ reportable by quickest means (telephone)
	▶ submit online form immediately
	▶ submit a report within ten days
	▶ examples – collapse of scaffolding; the collapse, overturning or failure of any load-bearing part of lifts and lifting equipment; explosion or fire resulting in the suspension of normal working for more than 24 hours

Records must be kept of

▶ any **accident, occupational disease or dangerous occurrence** which requires reporting under RIDDOR; and
▶ any other occupational accident causing injuries that result in a worker being away from work or incapacitated for more than three consecutive days (over-three-day injuries do not have to be reported, unless the incapacitation period goes on to exceed seven days).

Compensation and insurance issues

▶ importance of documentation and records
▶ need for pre- and post-accident risk assessments
▶ impact of Woolf Report and documentation required to defend a civil claim.

1.6

Health and safety management systems 4 – Act

Learning outcomes

Explain the purpose of, and procedures for, health and safety auditing ☐

Explain the purpose of, and procedures for, regular reviews of health and safety performance ☐

🔑 Key revision points

The role of performance review and audit ☐

The meaning, scope and purpose of health and safety audit ☐

The advantages and disadvantages of internal and external audit ☐

The reasons for measuring and monitoring health and safety performance ☐

The role of standards in the monitoring process ☐

The role of Boards in performance review ☐

The measures to continually improve health and safety performance ☐

The final ACT steps in the health and safety management control cycle are auditing, performance review and continual improvement.

Health and safety auditing

Auditing – the independent collection of information on the efficiency, effectiveness and reliability of the whole health and safety management system measured against specific standards. It will check that the following are in place:

▶ appropriate management arrangements;
▶ adequate risk control systems exist and implemented;
▶ appropriate workplace precautions; and
▶ appropriate documentation and records.

Audits should take place at regular intervals (every two to four years).

Other issues with audits

External audits:

▶ are independent of organisation;
▶ are competent;
▶ are familiar with external benchmarks;
▶ will not be inhibited from criticising members of management or the workforce;
▶ are more likely to be up to date with legal requirements and best practice in other companies;
▶ may be unfamiliar with the industry and seek unrealistic standards;
▶ are unlikely to be familiar with the workplace, tasks and processes;
▶ are more expensive than internal audits; and
▶ can offer bland reports.

Internal audits:

▶ are not independent of organisation and partiality may be questioned;
▶ may be subject to pressure from management and the workforce;
▶ usually require audit training;
▶ are less expensive than external audits;
▶ know the organisation well, particularly critical areas;
▶ likely to be aware of what is practicable for the industry;
▶ the ability to see improvements or a deterioration from the last audit;
▶ are familiar with the workforce and an individual's qualities and attitude;
▶ can spread good practice around the organisation; and
▶ may be unaware of external benchmarks.

Review of health and safety performance

Performance review is the final stage of the management process and reviews:

▶ all monitoring, inspection and audit reports;
▶ the adequacy of the health and safety management system, and performance standards, against external benchmarks;

▶ whether new legislation or guidance has been applied;

▶ whether the health and safety policy objectives have been met or need modification to ensure continuous improvement; and

▶ whether there has been adequate feedback to/from managers.

Reviews should aim to include:

▶ evaluation of compliance with legal and organisational requirements;

▶ incident data, recommendations and action plans from investigations;

▶ inspections, surveys, tours and sampling;

▶ absences and sickness records and their analysis;

▶ any reports on quality assurance or environmental protection;

▶ audit results and implementation;

▶ monitoring of data, reports and records;

▶ communications from enforcing authorities and insurers;

▶ any developments in legal requirements or best practice within the industry;

▶ changed circumstances or processes;

▶ benchmarking with other similar organisations;

▶ complaints from neighbours, customers and the public;

▶ effectiveness of consultation and internal communications;

▶ whether health and safety objectives have been met; and

▶ whether actions from previous reviews have been completed.

The Board should review health and safety performance at least once a year. The review process should:

▶ examine whether the health and safety policy requires revision;

▶ examine whether risk management and other health and safety issues have been effectively reported to the Board;

▶ report health and safety shortcomings;

▶ address any weaknesses with effective measures and develop a system to monitor their implementation; and

▶ undertake immediate reviews in the light of major shortcomings or events.

Continual improvement

Continual improvement of safety performance will be achieved through:

▶ active and reactive evaluations of facilities, equipment, documentation and procedures through safety audits and surveys;

▶ active evaluation of each individuals performance to verify the fulfilment of their safety responsibilities; and

▶ a reactive evaluation in order to verify the effectiveness of the system for control and mitigation of risk.

Measures that could be used to improve safety management include:

▶ more succinct procedures;

▶ improved safety reviews, studies and audits;

▶ improved reporting and analysis tools;

▶ improved hazards identification and risk assessment processes and improved awareness of risks in the organisation;

▶ improved relations with the subcontractors, suppliers and customers regarding safety;

▶ improved communication processes, including feedback from the personnel.

Unit FC1

Fire safety and risk management

2.1

Managing fire safety

Outline the moral, legal and financial consequences of inadequate management of fire safety	☐
Outline the legal framework for the regulation of fire safety in new, altered and existing buildings (including government guidance)	☐
Describe the roles and powers of enforcement agencies and other external agencies in relation to fire safety	☐
Outline the key features of a fire safety policy	☐
Outline the main sources of external fire safety information and the principles of their application	☐
Explain the purpose of, and the procedures for, investigating fires in the workplace	☐
Explain the legal and organisational requirements for recording and reporting fire related incidents	☐

Outline the moral, legal and financial consequences of inadequate management of fire safety

> ## Key revision points
>
> ▶ The size of the fire safety 'problem' in terms of the numbers of fire-related fatalities and injuries and environmental damage
> ▶ The duty of care owed by the occupier of a building
> ▶ Costs of inadequate management of fire safety including loss of business continuity
> ▶ Financial implications of false alarms (such as possible penalties that may be imposed, business interruption, etc.).

The potential consequences of a fire or the inadequate management of fire safety could include:

Moral/human harm

Those affected could include those in the premises and the surrounding area. The results could be:

▶ death;
▶ personal injury; and/or
▶ ill health.

In 2014–15 there were 258 fire fatalities and 3,235 non-fatal fire hospital casualties in England.[1]

Fires, worldwide, have caused major loss of life. These include:

1911	New York, USA	146 killed in a fire in a garment factory
1960	Busan, South Korea	68 killed in a fire in a rubber manufacturing factory
1988	Piper Alpha, UK, North Sea	167 killed by a fire on an oil platform
1993	Fujian, China	61 killed in a fire in a garment factory
1993	Shenzhen, China	81 killed in a fire in a toy factory
1993	Nakhon Pathom, Thailand	188 killed in a fire in a toy factory

2004	Rosepark Nursing Home, Scotland	14 elderly residents died
2006	Dhaka, Bangladesh	54 killed and 100 injured in a fire in a garment factory
2008	Casablanca, Morocco	55 killed in a fire in a furniture factory
2010	Heilongjiang, China	19 killed and 153 injured in an explosion at a firework factory
2012	Rayong, Thailand	12 killed and 100 injured in an explosion at a synthetic rubber factory
2012	Karachi, Pakistan	289 killed in a fire in a garments factory

Worldwide workplace fires causing loss of life[2]

UK major fires include:

▶ Great Fire of London, 1666
▶ Empire Palace Theatre, Edinburgh, 1911
▶ Henderson's Department Store, Liverpool, 1960
▶ Summerland Leisure Complex, Isle of Man, 1973
▶ Woolworths, Manchester, 1979
▶ Stardust Discotheque, Dublin, 1981
▶ Piper Alpha, UK, North Sea, 1983
▶ Bradford Football Stadium, 1985
▶ King's Cross Underground Station, 1987
▶ Littlewoods Department Store, Chesterfield, 1993
▶ The Conoco Philips Humber Refinery, 2001
▶ Buncefield, Hemel Hempstead, 2015.

Extra study

Look up these famous fires – what happened and why?

Legal implications

Those who are responsible for premises could potentially be liable for:

▶ prosecutions, including fines and imprisonment, brought by the Fire Authorities;

▶ prosecutions, including fines and imprisonment, brought by the Environmental Agencies; and

▶ civil cases being brought by those effected.

Persons responsible

The person responsible for fire safety is dependent upon which legislation applies. However, it is normally the person in charge of the premises and/or landlord – for example, the employer. They are known as:

▶ **'Responsible Person'** in England, under Regulatory Reform Fire Safety Order 2005

▶ **'Duty Holder'** in Scotland, under Fire Safety (Scotland) Regulations 2006

▶ **'Appropriate Person'** in Northern Ireland, Fire Safety Regulations (Northern Ireland) 2010.

Financial/economic implications

A fire at premises could result in:

▶ loss of business continuity;

▶ property damage;

▶ product damage;

▶ loss of business; and

▶ transport disruption in the area.

The loss of business continuity can affect staff, customers, the wider community and the economy. Many businesses affected by a major fire close and do not reopen.

An additional financial implication is the result of false alarms. In England, 2014–15, 44% of all incidents attended by local authority fire and rescue services were fire false alarms.[3] Possible causes of false alarms include:

▶ clandestine smoking;

▶ dust from maintenance;

▶ failure to isolate a zone in the vicinity of hot work;

▶ faults due to corrosion;
▶ horseplay;
▶ product spillage activating an optical detector;
▶ wiring defects;
▶ wrong choice of detector heads; and
▶ wrong positioning of detectors or call points.

Environmental factors

The result of a fire will, potentially, have a detrimental impact on the environment including:

▶ aesthetics – i.e. damaging the view;
▶ agricultural impact;
▶ air pollution;
▶ causing harm to flora and fauna;
▶ land/soil contamination;
▶ water pollution; and
▶ wildlife death and disturbance.

Revision exercise

Give TWO examples, for the following factors, that would be a consequence of inadequate management of fire safety:

(a) **Moral (2 examples)**
(b) **Legal (2)**
(c) **Financial (2)**
(d) **Environmental (2)**

Exam tip

You will not be expected to remember any specific fire incident and/or its details.

Outline the legal framework for the regulation of fire safety in new, altered and existing buildings (including government guidance)

> ## Key revision points
>
> ▶ UK Legislation
> ▶ Guidance documents
> ▶ Meaning of, and duties of, 'responsible person'
> ▶ Absolute and qualified duties: 'reasonably practicable'.

UK Legislation

UK Legislation, with regard to fire safety, is split dependent upon which country the premises are based in. In 2005 Fire Authorities (local Fire Brigade) discontinued issuing Fire Certificates to premises. The focus became the enforcement of fire safety. The approach towards fire safety, from the context of the Fire Safety Officers (inspectors), is General Fire Safety – i.e. raising the alarm and ensuring means of escape for those within the premises, which includes maintenance of the fire alarm and detection systems, etc. Fire Safety Audits are carried out by the inspectors using Chief Fire Officers' Association (CFOA) *Fire Safety Guidance Notes and Audit*.[4]

England and Wales

▶ Regulatory Reform Fire Safety Order 2005
▶ Fire and Rescue Services Act 2004
▶ The person responsible for fire safety is called the **'Responsible Person'.**

Scotland

▶ Fire Safety (Scotland) Regulations 2006
▶ Fire (Scotland) Act 2005
▶ The person responsible for fire safety is called the **'Duty Holder'.**

Northern Ireland

▶ Fire and Rescue Services (Northern Ireland) Order 2006
▶ Fire Safety Regulations (Northern Ireland) 2010
▶ The person responsible for fire safety is called the **'Appropriate Person'.**

Guidance documents

Guidance documents used for Fire Safety include:

Department for Communities and Local Government (DCLG 2005) Fire Guides,[5] Fire safety in:

▶ *offices and shops;*
▶ *factories and warehouses;*
▶ *premises providing sleeping accommodation;*
▶ *premises providing residential care;*
▶ *educational premises;*
▶ *small and medium places of assembly (up to 300 people);*
▶ *large places of assembly (over 300 people);*
▶ *theatres and cinemas;*
▶ *open air events and venues;*
▶ *healthcare premises;*
▶ *the transport premises and facilities;*
▶ *stables and agricultural premises; and*
▶ *means of escape for disabled people.*

These guides are freely available at https://www.gov.uk/government/collections/fire-safety-law-and-guidance-documents-for-business.

Whether you are undertaking a fire risk assessment or managing the fire safety of premises, the above guidelines are invaluable.

Exercise

Download the relevant guide for your workplace, and view this against the current fire risk assessment and fire safety policy.

Meaning of, and duties of, 'responsible person' and meaning of 'relevant persons'

The meaning of the 'Responsible Person' is defined, within the Regulatory Reform Fire Safety Order 2005, as:[6]

(a) in relation to a workplace, the employer, if the workplace is to any extent under his control;

(b) in relation to any premises not falling within paragraph (a) –

    (i) the person who has control of the premises (as occupier or otherwise) in connection with the carrying on by him of a trade, business or other undertaking (for profit or not); or

    (ii) the owner, where the person in control of the premises does not have control in connection with the carrying on by that person of a trade, business or other undertaking.

A **relevant person** is defined as:

▶ any person (including the responsible person) who is or may be lawfully on the premises;

▶ any person in the immediate vicinity of the premises who is at risk from a fire on the premises;

▶ but does not include a fire-fighter who is carrying out his duties in relation to a function of a fire and rescue authority.

Absolute and qualified duties

With regards to the duty to take general fire precautions the responsible person must:

▶ take such general fire precautions as will ensure, so far as is reasonably practicable, the safety of any of his employees;

▶ in relation to relevant persons who are not his employees, take such general fire precautions as may reasonably be required in the circumstances of the case to ensure that the premises are safe.

Onus of proving limits of what is practicable or reasonably practicable:

▶ In any proceedings for an offence under local legislation consisting of a failure to comply with a duty or requirement so far as is practicable or so far as is reasonably practicable, it is for the accused to prove that it was not practicable or reasonably practicable to do more than was in fact done to satisfy the duty or requirement.

There are three levels of statutory duty placed on the responsible person:

▶ **Absolute Duty**. No assessment of risk is required, but the duty is absolute, and the employer has no choice but to undertake the duty. For example, verbs used in the regulations will include 'must' and 'shall'.

▶ **Practicable**. This means that if the duty is technically possible or feasible, then it must be done irrespective of any difficulty, inconvenience or cost.

▶ **Reasonably Practicable**. This duty requires a risk assessment to be undertaken – for example, if the risk of injury is low compared to the cost (money), time, inconvenience and effort required to reduce the risk, then no action is necessary.

Revision exercise

Identify Fire Guides, published by the Department for Communities and Local Government. (8)

Exam tip

Learn the name of ALL the above guides!

Describe the roles and powers of enforcement agencies and other external agencies in relation to fire safety

Key revision points

▶ The roles and powers of enforcement agencies and other external agencies in relation to fire safety
▶ The powers of inspectors under local legislation

> ▶ The powers of authorised officers under local legislation
> ▶ Enforcement; notices (alterations, enforcement, prohibition); conditions for serving; effects; procedures; rights and effects of appeal; role of magistrates court; and penalties for failure to comply.

The roles and powers of enforcement agencies and other external agencies in relation to fire safety

Inspectors will undertake a fire safety audit on premises. The audit will address issues with regard to the protection of life, rather than addressing issues such as the environment, business continuity, property and product protection.

With regard to life safety, the result of the audit will state if the premises is:

- ▶ broadly compliant;
- ▶ non-compliant – with minor deficiencies; or
- ▶ non-compliant – with major deficiencies.

Inspectors have various options available to them:

- ▶ Informal action – verbal and/or written
- ▶ Formal action – alterations notice
- ▶ Formal action – enforcement notice
- ▶ Formal action – prohibition notice
- ▶ Court action – prosecution and/or imprisonment.

Fire inspectors may be granted specific powers under local legislation:

- ▶ To enter any premises.
- ▶ To inspect the whole or part of the premises and anything in them.
- ▶ To identify the responsible person in relation to the premises.
- ▶ To require the production of any records relating to fire safety.
- ▶ To inspect and take copies of, or of any entry in, the records.

▶ To require any person having responsibilities in relation to any premises provide information in relation to fire safety.

▶ To give him/her such facilities and assistance with respect to any matters or things to which the responsibilities of that person extend as are necessary.

▶ To take samples of any articles or substances found in any premises.

▶ In the case of any article or substance found in any premises which he/she has power to enter, being an article or substance which appears to him/her to have caused or to be likely to cause danger to the safety of relevant persons, to cause it to be dismantled or subjected to any process or test (but not so as to damage or destroy it unless this is, in the circumstances, necessary).

The powers of authorised officers under the local legislation includes:

An employee of a fire and rescue authority who is authorised in writing by the authority – i.e. authorised officer – can (if the officer reasonably believes a fire to have broken out or to be about to break out, or a road traffic accident to have occurred, or an emergency of another kind to have occurred):

▶ enter premises or a place, by force if necessary, without the consent of the owner or occupier of the premises or place;

▶ move or break into a vehicle without the consent of its owner;

▶ close a highway;

▶ stop and regulate traffic;

▶ restrict the access of persons to premises or a place.

Enforcement notices (alterations, enforcement, prohibition) may be served

Alterations notice

This requires the responsible person to notify the fire and rescue authority of any proposed changes which may increase the risk in the premises. They are issued where a fire and rescue authority considers that the premises constitute a serious risk or may constitute a risk if changes are made. An alterations notice does not mean that the responsible person has failed to comply with local legislation.

Enforcement notice

This is issued where the responsible person has failed to comply with local legislation and details corrective measures that the person is legally obliged to complete within a set timescale, to comply with the law.

Prohibition notice

This is issued where the use of the premises may constitute an imminent risk of death or serious injury to the persons using them. This may be a restriction of use (for example, imposing a maximum number of persons allowed in the premises) or a prohibition of a specific use of all or part of the premises (for example, prohibiting the use of specific floors or rooms for sleeping accommodation).

In certain circumstances a fire and rescue authority will prosecute individuals and companies for breaches of legislation. In the UK, a sentence of two years imprisonment and/or an unlimited fine per individual offence is the maximum sentence available to the courts.

It is possible to appeal against an enforcement and/or alterations notice. This will suspend the enforcement notice until the appeal has been finally disposed of, or withdrawal of the appeal. The prohibition notice will remain in force during the appeal unless the court directs the suspending of the notice.

Three possible outcomes from an appeal:

▶ The notice may be cancelled – (the notice is not enforced).
▶ The notice may be affirmed – (must be complied with).
▶ The notice may be affirmed with modifications – (comply with the amended version).

Revision exercise

Identify FOUR powers an inspector may use. (4)

Identify FOUR powers an officer may use. (4)

Exam tip

If you were asked to IDENTIFY THREE Enforcement Notices, then your answer would simply need to be:

(1) Alterations notice
(2) Enforcement notice
(3) Prohibition notice

to gain the marks.

Outline the key features of a fire safety policy

Key revision points

Responsibility for fire safety within an organisation and the arrangements for ensuring fire safety to include arrangements for:

▶ planning
▶ organisation
▶ control
▶ monitoring
▶ review
▶ arrangements for vulnerable people
▶ degraded systems planning.

An appropriate fire protection policy for the company should include[7]

(1) Active leadership for fire protection issues;
(2) Management of fire protection;
(3) Plans for training in fire protection;
(4) Fire protection rules;
(5) A description of fire protection;
(6) Operating and maintenance instructions for fire protection;

(7) A control system for fire protection; and

(8) Monitoring procedures for fire protection.

Developing a fire safety policy

A specific fire safety policy can be developed to manage fire safety. This will outline those responsible for fire safety and their roles and responsibilities. It will also address specific fire safety arrangements.

Fire safety policy headings

The following headings may be considered when developing a fire safety policy.

Statement of intent/introduction

The aim of a fire safety policy is to reduce the risk and minimise the occurrence of a fire within. It is also to minimise the impact of a fire on life safety, environment, business continuity, and property and product protection. Reference to legal compliance is also, normally, included in this section.

Roles and responsibilities

The specific roles and responsibilities are to be outlined. This may take the form of an organisation chart (organogram). Details for the following are likely to be included:

▶ Employer/Director

▶ Fire Safety Manager

▶ Fire Wardens (roles for both emergency and non-emergency situations)

▶ Other Relevant Persons (employees, etc.).

Arrangements

▶ **Fire Prevention** focuses on the three elements of the fire triangle (oxygen, ignition and fuel), with the aim of preventing them uniting.

▶ **Fire Precaution** focuses on reducing the risks to people from the result of a fire and smoke spread. It focuses on assessing means of escape; means of detection; maintenance of fire safety provisions; and management of fire safety.

Revision exercise

Identify FOUR persons who may be named in a fire safety policy and in each case **outline** their possible roles. (4)

Outline the main sources of external fire safety information and the principles of their application

---

Key revision points

▶ Appropriate national legislation and guidance such as the UK Department for Communities and Local Government practical fire safety guidance
▶ Fire guidance
▶ The principles of application of local guidance.

Guidance documents used for Fire Safety, as already mentioned above include:

Department for Communities and Local Government (DCLG 2005) Fire Guides[8] fire safety in:

▶ *offices and shops;* ①
▶ *factories and warehouses;* ②
▶ *premises providing sleeping accommodation;* ③
▶ *premises providing residential care;* ④
▶ *educational premises;* ⑤

▶ *small and medium places of assembly (up to 300 people);* (6)
▶ *large places of assembly (over 300 people);* (7)
▶ *theatres and cinemas;* (8)
▶ *open air events and venues;* (9)
▶ *healthcare premises;* (10)
▶ *the transport premises and facilities;* (11)
▶ *stables and agricultural premises; and* (12)
▶ *means of escape for disabled people.* (13)

Revision tip

Did you remember all these guides?

Further fire guidance includes:

Association of British Insurers

The Association of British Insurers represents the general insurance and long-term and investment savings industries. The Association was formed in 1985.

The Confederation of fire protection associations in Europe

CFPA-Europe is an association of national organisations in Europe concerned primarily with fire prevention and protection and also safety and security and other associated risks. There are over 30 guidance documents available.[9]

National fire protection association

The mission of the international non-profit NFPA, established in 1896, is to reduce the worldwide burden of fire and other hazards on the quality of life by providing and advocating consensus codes and standards, research, training and education.

British Standards Institute (BSI)

BSI is the business standards company that helps organisations make excellence a habit – all over the world. Their business is enabling others to perform better.

British Standards, relevant for fire safety include:[10]

▶ BS EN 7671:2008+A3:2015 Requirements for Electrical Installations, IET Wiring Regulations;

▶ BS EN 5266–1:2011 Emergency lighting;

▶ BS 5306–9:2015 for fire extinguishers service and maintenance;

▶ BS EN 5839–1:2013 Fire detection and fire alarm systems for buildings;

▶ BS EN 9999:2008 Code of practice for fire safety in the design, management; use of buildings, issued by the British Standards Institute; and

▶ BS EN 12845:2015 Fixed fire fighting systems, automatic sprinkler systems design, installation and maintenance.

Note: the above is not an exhaustive list.

It is important that fire safety professionals keep up to date with changes. For example, the new edition of BS 5306–9 brings together two standards, providing all the requirements for the installation and recharging of portable fire extinguishers. It directs building owners to ensure that there are effective fire fighting provisions in their buildings.

Other UK documents, relevant for fire safety, include:

▶ Approved Documents of the Building Regulations: Approved Document B – Fire Safety: Volume 1: Dwellinghouses;[11]

▶ Approved Documents of the Building Regulations: Approved Document B – Fire Safety: Volume 2: Buildings other than dwellinghouses;[12]

▶ Designing and Managing Against the Risk of Fire in Schools (BB100);[13]

▶ Fire safety in purpose-built blocks of flats;[14]

▶ Guidance on fire safety provisions for certain types of existing housing;[15]

▶ Health technical memorandum 05–02: Firecode guidance in support of functional provisions (fire safety in the design of healthcare premises), 2015;[16]

▶ Institution of Engineering and Technology (2012) Code of Practice for in-service inspection and testing of electrical equipment 4th Edition. London: IET;[17]

▶ A guide to reducing the number of false alarms from fire-detection and fire-alarm systems;[18]

▶ Arson: a call to action A 'State of the Nation' Report. Arson Prevention Forum;[19]

▶ Standard Fire Precautions for Contractors Engaged on Crown Works;[20]

▶ Fire Prevention on Construction Sites;[21] and

▶ Fire Safety in Construction Work.[22]

PAS (Publicly Available Specification) documents:

PAS79:2012: *PAS79:2012 Fire Risk Assessment. Guidance and a Recommended Methodology* gives guidance and corresponding examples of documentation for undertaking, and recording the significant findings of, fire risk assessments in premises and parts of premises for which fire risk assessments are required by legislation. It is not applicable in the case of a single-family private dwelling, or necessarily applicable to premises during the construction phase but is applicable to vacant premises, for which a fire risk assessment is required. The methodology is intended to provide a structured approach to fire risk assessment for people with knowledge of the principles of fire safety; it is not intended as a guide to fire safety.

Revision exercise

Identify documents that could be used when developing a fire safety policy. (8)

Exam tip

The above mock question links the last two learning outcomes together.

If you were identifying documents the specific number will not be required to gain the mark.

Explain the purpose of, and the procedures for, investigating fires in the workplace

---

Key revision points

▶ Purpose of investigating fires in the workplace
▶ Basic fire-related investigation procedures – procedural differences and definitions (e.g. fatal and non-fatal fires, accidental or arson fires and false alarms)
▶ Investigation preparation, preserving the fire scene
▶ Liaison and working protocols with the police and other external agencies
▶ Identify the underlying causes of the fire
▶ Remedial actions to prevent recurrence.

Reasons for investigating fires in the work place

After the event of a fire it is essential that the causes of the incident are investigated. In particular:

▶ The need to determine the origin of the fire;
▶ The need to develop and introduce the appropriate remedial measures to prevent recurrence;
▶ To determine the effectiveness of procedures currently in place and to develop new arrangements if they are found to be deficient;

▶ To allay concerns of possible damage to the environment;

▶ To assess damage and gather evidence for insurance claim;

▶ To determine whether there has been a breach of legal requirements and to gather evidence to defend any possible criminal or civil proceedings which might be taken;

▶ To determine whether there has been a fault or failure by an individual or individuals which could lead to disciplinary action being taken;

▶ To identify if a crime has been committed (i.e. arson) and to possibly cover up another crime;

▶ To identify possible trends;

▶ To reassure stakeholders such as financial institutions, insurance companies and the general public;

▶ To verify insurance claims.

The results of the investigation and the effects and consequences are of great importance to owners of the premises, fire and rescue authorities, insurers, etc. In the case of a serious fire in the workplace, it is inevitable that the fire and rescue authority will conduct its own investigation, in order to detect the persons responsible.

Categories of fires[23]

The three categories of fires are:

1 **Primary fires:** fires with one or more of the following characteristics:
   ▶ all fires in buildings and vehicles that are not derelict or in outdoor structures
   ▶ any fires involving casualties or rescues
   ▶ any fire attended by five or more appliances.

2 **Secondary fires:** the majority of outdoor fires including grassland and refuse fires, unless these involve casualties, rescues or property loss or unless five or more appliances attend. It includes fires in derelict buildings.

3 **Chimney fires:** fires in buildings where the flame was contained within the chimney structure and did not involve casualties, rescues or attendance by five or more pumping appliances.

Stages of an investigation

Fire investigations are likely to utilise the following stages:

1 Gather factual information
2 Analyse the information
3 Identify controls
4 Plan remedial action.

Accidental fires

Main causes of accidental fires:

▶ faulty appliances and leads;
▶ misuse of equipment or appliances;
▶ smoking materials;
▶ candles;
▶ chip/fat pan and other cooking appliances;
▶ playing with fire; and
▶ placing articles too close to heat source.

Deliberate fires

Main causes of fires started deliberately (arson/wilful fire-raising) include:

▶ pyromania;
▶ to conceal a crime;
▶ insurance claim;
▶ disgruntled employee;
▶ disagreeing with policy of organisation (e.g. animal testing labs);
▶ wanting to see fire engines or fire officers tackling a fire; etc.

False alarms

These are events in which the Fire and Rescue Service believes they are called to a reportable fire and then find there is no incident. False alarms are categorised as follows:

▶ **Malicious False Alarms** are calls made with the intention of getting the fire and rescue service to attend a non-existent fire-related event, including deliberate and suspected malicious intentions.

▶ **Good Intent False Alarms** are calls made in good faith in the belief that the fire and rescue service really would attend a fire.

▶ **False Alarms** Malfunctioning of fire alarm systems or accidental initiation of alarm apparatus by persons.

Revision exercise

Outline reasons to investigate fires that occur in the workplace. (8)

Exam tip

Outline answers are generally short sentences – an example of a possible answer (for ONE MARK) to the above question would be either:

the need to develop and introduce the appropriate remedial measures to prevent recurrence

or

to determine the effectiveness of procedures currently in place and to develop new arrangements if they are found to be deficient.

However, to simply write

prevent fire

is unlikely to gain any marks.

Explain the legal and organisational requirements for recording and reporting fire related incidents

Key revision points

▶ The need for processes and procedures for the recording and reporting of fire-related injuries, fatalities and dangerous occurrences in the workplace

▶ Process and procedures for recording and reporting fire related fatalities, major injuries or dangerous occurrences

▶ Examples of typical records: accident book; fire logbook; general incident or occurrence book; and appropriate forms (such as) F2508

▶ Use and review of fire risk assessments.

Processes and procedures for the recording and reporting of fire-related injuries

In the UK, under the Reporting of Injuries, Diseases and Dangerous Occurrences Regulations (RIDDOR) 2013,[24] several types of dangerous occurrence require reporting in circumstances where the incident has the potential to cause injury or death.

The list of 'specified injuries' in RIDDOR 2013 replaces the previous list of 'major injuries' in RIDDOR 1995. *Specified injuries* are (regulation 4):

▶ fractures, other than to fingers, thumbs and toes
▶ amputations
▶ any injury likely to lead to permanent loss of sight or reduction in sight
▶ any crush injury to the head or torso causing damage to the brain or internal organs

► serious burns (including scalding) which
  ▷ cover more than 10% of the body
  ▷ cause significant damage to the eyes, respiratory system or other vital organs

► any scalping requiring hospital treatment
► any loss of consciousness caused by head injury or asphyxia
► any other injury arising from working in an enclosed space which
  ▷ leads to hypothermia or heat-induced illness
  ▷ requires resuscitation or admittance to hospital for more than 24 hours.

Explosion or fire

Any unintentional explosion or fire in any plant or premises which results in the stoppage of that plant, or the suspension of normal work in those premises, for more than 24 hours.

Responsible persons should complete the appropriate online report form listed below. The form will then be submitted directly to the RIDDOR database. The online form **F2508DOE** is available at https://extranet.hse.gov.uk/lfserver/external/**F2508DOE**.

Records

Examples of typical records that would be used for fire safety may include:

► Accident book.
► Fire logbook (which is likely to contain details of):
  ▷ weekly fire alarm tests;
  ▷ monthly emergency lighting tests;
  ▷ monthly fire fighting equipment user checks;
  ▷ monthly fire door checks;
  ▷ additional fire safety checks;
  ▷ fire instruction and staff training record;
  ▷ fire incidents log;
  ▷ details of fire drills;
  ▷ details of fire and rescue authority visits; and
  ▷ reference information.

▶ General incident or occurrence book.
▶ Appropriate country specific forms – for example, F2508.

Use and review of fire risk assessments

Within local legislation there is normally requirement for the Responsible Person (normally the person in charge of the premises and/or landlord) to have a fire risk assessment undertaken. Regulatory Reform Fire Safety Order 2005, Article 9(1), states:

> *The responsible person must make a suitable and sufficient assessment of the risks to which relevant persons are exposed for the purpose of identifying the general fire precautions he needs to take to comply with the requirements and prohibitions imposed on him by or under this Order.*[25]

A suitable and sufficient risk assessment should:

▶ *identify the significant risks and ignore the trivial ones;*
▶ *identify and prioritize the measures required to comply with any relevant statutory provisions;*
▶ *remain appropriate to the nature of the work and valid over a reasonable period of time;*
▶ *identify the risk arising from or in connection with the work. The level of detail should be proportionate to the risk.*

The significant findings that should be recorded include a detailed statement of the hazards and risks, the preventative, [sic] protective or control measures in place and any further measures required to reduce the risks present.[26]

Reasons to review a fire risk assessment may include:

▶ Change in legislation
▶ Change in guidance/British Standards
▶ After a fire
▶ After a false alarm/number of false alarms
▶ Change in procedures
▶ Change in equipment
▶ Change in premises

▶ Change in number staff
▶ If there are now venerable employees/visitors to premises
▶ Passage of time – i.e. one year
▶ Requests from insurers
▶ Requests from fire and rescue authority.

Revision exercise

Identify the possible details recorded in a fire logbook. (6)

Exam tip

The above question is an IDENTIFY, so a simple list of the records is all that would be required to gain the marks – for example:

▶ Weekly fire alarm tests.

References

1 Available at: https://www.gov.uk/government/uploads/system/uploads/attachment_data/file/456623/Fire_Statistics_Monitor_April_2014_to_March_2015_Updated260815.pdf

2 Available at: http://www.ilo.org/wcmsp5/groups/public/—ed_protect/—protrav/—safework/documents/publication/wcms_194781.pdf with additional information added from http://www.bbc.co.uk/news/uk-scotland-glasgow-west-13132557

3 Available at: https://www.gov.uk/government/uploads/system/uploads/attachment_data/file/456623/Fire_Statistics_Monitor_April_2014_to_March_2015_Updated260815.pdf

4 Chief Fire Officers Association (CFOA) (2009a) *Revised Fire Safety Guidance Notes and Audit Form Version 4.2*. Chief Fire Officers Association. Available at: http://www.cfoa.org.uk/download/12191

5 Department for Communities and Local Government Fire Guides Available at: https://www.gov.uk/government/collections/fire-safety-law-and-guidance-documents-for-business

6 Great Britain (2005) *Regulatory Reform (Fire Safety) Order 2005*. London: The Stationery Office. Available at: http://www.legislation.gov.uk/uksi/2005/1541/pdfs/uksi_20051541_en.pdf

7 Available at: http://www.cfpa-e.eu/files/CFPA_E_Guideline_No_1_2002.pdf

8 Department for Communities and Local Government Fire Guides Available at: https://www.gov.uk/government/collections/fire-safety-law-and-guidance-documents-for-business

9 Available at: http://www.cfpa-e.eu/cfpa-e-guidelines/guidelines-fire-protection/

   31:2013 Protection against self-ignition and explosions in handling and storage of silage and fodder in farms
   30:2013 Managing fire safety of historic buildings
   29:2013 Protection of paintings: transport, exhibition and storage
   28:2012 Fire safety in laboratories
   27:2011 Fire safety in apartment buildings
   26:2010 Fire protection of temporary buildings on construction sites
   25:2010 Emergency plan
   24:2010 Fire safe homes
   23:2010 Securing the operational readiness of fire control systems
   22:2012 Wind turbines – Fire protection guideline
   21:2012 Fire Prevention on Construction Sites
   20:2012 Fire Safety in Camping Sites
   19:2009 Fire Safety Engineering concerning Evacuation from Buildings
   18:2013 Fire protection on chemical manufacturing sites
   17:2008 Fire safety in farm buildings
   16:2008 Fire protection in offices
   15:2012 Fire safety in guest harbours and marinas
   14:2007 Fire protection in information technology facilities
   13:2006 Fire protection documentation
   12:2012 Fire safety basics for hot work operatives
   11:2005 Recommended numbers of fire protection trained staff
   10:2008 Smoke alarms in the home
    9:2012 Fire safety in restaurants
    8:2004 Prevention arson – information to young people
    7:2011 Safety distance between waste containers and buildings
    6:2011 Fire safety in residential homes for the elderly
    5:2003 Guidance signs, emergency lighting and general lighting
    4:2010 Introduction to qualitative fire risk assessment
    3:2011 Certification of thermographers
    2:2013 Panic and emergency exit devices
    1:2002 Internal fire protection control

10 British Standards Available at: http://shop.bsigroup.com/Navigate-by/Standards/

11 DCLG (2013) *Approved Documents of the Building Regulations: Approved Document B – Fire Safety: Volume 1: Dwellinghouses*. Available at: http://www.planningportal.gov.uk/uploads/br/BR_PDF_AD_B1_2013.pdf

12 DCLG (2013) *Approved Documents of the Building Regulations: Approved Document B – Fire Safety: Volume 2: Buildings Other Than Dwellinghouses*. Available at: http://www.planningportal.gov.uk/uploads/br/BR_PDF_AD_B2_2013.pdf

13 DfES (2005) *BB100: Designing and Managing Against the Risk of Fire in Schools*. Available at: https://www.education.gov.uk/consultations/downloadableDocs/BB100%20July%2005%20-%20Complete.pdf

14 Local Government Association (2012) *Fire Safety in Purpose-Built Blocks of Flats*. Available at: http://www.local.gov.uk/c/document_library/get_file?uuid=1138bf70–2e50–400c-bf81–9a3c4dbd6575

15 LACORS (2008) Guidance on Fire Safety Provisions for Certain Types of Existing Housing. Available at: http://www.cieh.org/library/Knowledge/Housing/National_fire_safety_guidance_08.pdf

16 Health technical memorandum 05–02: Firecode guidance in support of functional provisions (fire safety in the design of healthcare premises), 2015. Available at: https://www.gov.uk/government/uploads/system/uploads/attachment_data/file/473012/HTM_05–02_2015.pdf

17 Institution of Engineering and Technology (2012) *Code of Practice for In-Service Inspection and Testing of Electrical Equipment*, 4th edn. London: IET. Available at: http://electrical.theiet.org/books/inspection-test/in-service-inspection-4th-ed.cfm

18 ODPM (2012) *A Guide to Reducing the Number of False Alarms from Fire-Detection and Fire-Alarm Systems*. Available at: http://www.nifrs.org/wp-content/uploads/2012/05/A-guide-to-reducing-the-number-of-false-alarms-from-fire-detection-and-fire-alarm-systems.pdf

19 Arson Prevention Forum (2014) *Arson: A Call to Action A 'State of the Nation' Report*. Available at: http://www.stoparsonuk.org/documents/resources/DS2014–1156ArsonReportandappendix.pdf

20 HMSO (2005) *Standard Fire Precautions for Contractors Engaged on Crown Works*. Available at: http://regulations.completepicture.co.uk/pdf/Fire/Standard%20fire%20precautions%20for%20contractors%20engaged%20on%20Crown%20works.%20applicable%20to%20.pdf

21 Fire Protection Association (2015) *Fire Prevention on Construction Sites*. Available at: http://www.thefpa.co.uk/shop/shop_product_details.380EF9C6-D3F1–49FB-8BBAA662A9386E29.html?shop_category=

22 HSE (2010) *Fire Safety in Construction*. Available at: http://www.hse.gov.uk/pubns/books/hsg168.htm

23 Available at: https://www.gov.uk/government/uploads/system/uploads/attachment_data/file/275224/Fire_Statistics_Monitor_April_2013_to_September_2013__final_.pdf p15

24 RIDDOR (2013) Schedule 2, Part 1. Available at: http://www.legislation.gov.uk/uksi/2013/1471/schedule/2/made

25 Great Britain (2005) *Regulatory Reform (Fire Safety) Order 2005*. London: The Stationery Office. Available at: http://www.legislation.gov.uk/uksi/2005/1541/pdfs/uksi_20051541_en.pdf

26 Hughes, P. and Ferret, E. (2011) *Introduction to Health and Safety at Work*, 5th edn. Oxford: Taylor and Francis. p.101.

2.2

Principles of fire and explosion

Learning outcomes

Explain the principles of the combustion process in relation to fire safety

Explain the principles and conditions for the ignition of solids, liquids and gases

Identify the classification of fires

Describe the principles of fire growth and fire spread

Outline the principles of explosion and explosive combustion

Explain the principles of the combustion process in relation to fire safety

The fire triangle principle illustrates that to start a fire the three components need to be present, and a chemical reaction needs to take place:

▶ ignition source;
▶ fuel; and
▶ oxygen.

NOTE: below (methods of preventing or controlling ignition of combustible materials in relation to their properties) identifies examples of each headings of the fire triangle.

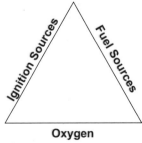

Oxygen

Figure 3 The fire triangle

Preventing the three elements of the fire triangle from uniting will stop the fire occurring in the first place.

By removing any one of the flowing components, the fire will cease:

▶ heat;
▶ fuel; and
▶ oxygen.

Revision exercise

Identify the **THREE** components that make up the fire triangle. (3)

Exam tip

Whilst it is not a requirement to draw your answers, if you want to you could, for example, include the fire triangle in your answer.

Explain the principles and conditions for the ignition of solids, liquids and gases

---

Key revision points

▶ Meaning and relevance of flash point, fire point and ignition point (kindling point); auto ignition temperature; vapour density; vapour pressure; flammable; highly flammable; upper flammable limit; lower flammable limit; combustion
▶ The conditions required to cause the ignition of combustible solids, flammable liquids and gaseous materials
▶ The methods of preventing or controlling ignition of combustible solid and flammable liquid and gaseous materials in relation to their physical and chemical properties
▶ The properties and safe storage of liquefied petroleum gas (LPG).

Fire terminology used in fire safety

▶ **Flash point** – the lowest temperature at which there is sufficient vaporisation of a substance capable of producing a flash momentarily when a heat source is applied.

▶ **Fire point** – lowest temperature at which the application of an ignition source will lead to continued burning.

▶ **Ignition point** (kindling point) / ignition temperature – lowest temperature of a heated surface at which, under specified conditions, the ignition of a flammable gas or vapour in contact with the surface will occur.

▶ **Auto ignition temperature** – lowest temperature at which a flammable gas/vapour-air mixture will ignite from its own heat source or contact with a heated surface without needing a spark or flame.

▶ **Vapour density** – the weight of a vapour or gas compared to an equal volume of air (air = 1). If greater than 1.0, the vapour or gas is heavier than air and will concentrate in the low places.

▶ **Vapour pressure** – the pressure of a vapour in contact with its liquid or solid form – i.e. tendency for a solid or liquid to evaporate into the air. The lower the boiling point, the higher the vapour pressure.

▶ **Category 1: Extremely flammable liquid and vapour** – Flash point < 23°C and initial boiling point ≤ 35°C

▶ **Category 2: Highly flammable liquid and vapour** – Flash point < 23°C and initial boiling point > 35°C

▶ **Category 3: Flammable liquid and vapour** – Flashpoint ≥ 23°C and ≤ 60°C

▶ **Category 4: Combustible liquid** – Flashpoint > 60°C and ≤ 93°C

▶ **Upper flammable limit** – highest concentration of a flammable substance in air within which a self-propagating flame can occur.

▶ **Lower flammable limit** – lowest concentration of a flammable substance in air within which a self-propagating flame can occur.

Conditions required that cause the ignition of combustible solids, flammable liquids and gaseous materials

By uniting the three elements of the fire triangle, a fire will occur.

▶ The presence of heat, whether from an external source, the exothermic nature of the combustion process or radiated from combustion products enables un-burnt fuel to be heated and ultimately ignited.

▶ Combustible fuel must be present, and its amount, chemical composition and physical state determines the susceptibility for the fire to continue.

▶ There must be a supply of oxygen whether from surrounding air or from oxidising agents or oxygen cylinders to react chemically with the fuel.

Chemistry of combustion

Combustion is a chemical reaction between substances, usually including oxygen and usually accompanied by the generation of heat and light in the form of flame.[1]

For example, when a match is struck, friction heats the head to a temperature at which the chemicals react and generate more heat than can escape into the air and therefore burns with a flame. The molecules in the matchstick break down and give off vapour causing more heat to be released, propagating further chemical reactions.

Complete and incomplete combustion (reaction)

There are two types of combustion: complete and incomplete combustion.

1 Complete combustion is when the substance is completely burned and only carbon dioxide and water remain. Complete combustion produces an orange or blue flame.

hydrocarbon + oxygen → carbon dioxide + water

2 Incomplete combustion occurs when there is not enough oxygen, or a high enough temperature, for the carbon to turn into carbon dioxide and therefore producing carbon monoxide. Incomplete combustion produces a yellow flame

hydrocarbon + oxygen → carbon monoxide + carbon + water

Endothermic and exothermic reactions

An **endothermic** reaction must absorb energy to proceed, normally from its surroundings. It cannot occur spontaneously, but, when the reaction absorbs energy, a drop in temperature is noted.

An **exothermic** reaction on the other hand is one that releases energy in the form of heat, light or sound. It can occur spontaneously, emitting heat to its surroundings causing an increase in temperature. Some exothermic reactions produce heat quickly and can cause explosions – for example, exothermic reaction of a substance with an oxidizer.

Oxidizer

A chemical that reacts with and gives off large amounts of oxygen, for example:

▶ Benzoyl peroxide;
▶ Bleach;
▶ Perchloric acid; and
▶ Peroxides (including Hydrogen peroxide).

Stages of combustion

The four stages of combustion are:

1 Induction;
2 Growth;
3 Steady state; and
4 Decay.

From **http://www.nist.gov/fire/fire_behavior.cfm.**

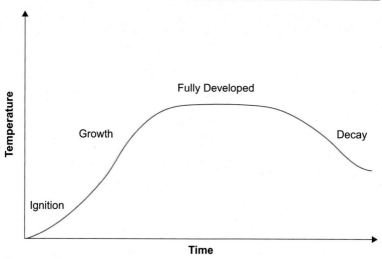

Figure 4 The stages of combustion

Methods of preventing or controlling ignition of combustible materials in relation to their properties

Fire prevention, which forms a significant part of the fire risk assessment, requires that ignition of combustible materials are controlled within the workplace.

The following are examples of possible ignition sources within the work place:[2]

▶ electrical sources of ignition;
▶ smoking;
▶ arson;
▶ portable heaters and heating installations;
▶ cooking;
▶ lightning;
▶ housekeeping;
▶ hazards introduced by outside contractors and building works;
▶ dangerous substances; and

119

▶ process fire hazards:

   ▷ hot work (welding, grinding, etc.);

   ▷ overheating of machinery; and

   ▷ spontaneous ignition of oil and solvent soaked materials.

The following are examples of possible fuel sources within the work place:

▶ paper and cardboard;

▶ furniture, fixtures and fittings;

▶ structural materials;

▶ wall and ceiling linings;

▶ flammable liquids;

▶ flammable gases (cylinders and piped gas);

▶ flammable vapours;

▶ combustible materials; and

▶ explosive materials.

The following are examples of possible oxygen sources within the work place:

▶ heating and ventilation Systems (HAVS);

▶ natural ventilation (from open windows);

▶ oxidizing materials;

▶ oxygen condensers; and

▶ oxygen cylinders.

Revision exercise

State the THREE components that make up the fire triangle. (3)
Describe the conditions required for the combustion process to be maintained. (5)

Exam tip

Fire terminology, above, could be used within exam questions. Do you know the difference between Flash Point and Fire Point?

Write these out until you don't need to read the definition anymore!

Identify the classification of fires

Key revision points

▶ The classification of fire according to its fuel source
▶ Properties and safe storage of liquefied petroleum gas (LPG).

Fire is classified in accordance with the types of fuel, for the UK:

Class A – Combustible solids, e.g. paper, textiles, wood, etc.

Class B – Flammable liquids

B1 (liquids soluble in water)

B2 (liquids not soluble in water)

Class C – Combustible gases

Class D – Combustible metals

Class F – Cooking oils or fats

NOTE: Electricity in not a class of fire, as it is not a fuel!

Different countries use different classification systems – for example, in the United States:

Class A – Combustible solids, e.g. paper, textiles, wood, etc.

Class B – Flammable liquids

Class C – Electrically energised equipment

Class E – Combustible metals

Class K – Cooking oils or fats

In Australia:

Class A – Combustible solids, e.g. paper, textiles, wood, etc.

Class B – Flammable liquids

Class C – Combustible gases

Class E – Electrically energised equipment

Class F – Cooking oils or fats

121

Properties and safe storage of liquefied petroleum gas (LPG)

LPG is used as a fuel in a range of applications including heating and cooking appliances, industrial applications, and in vehicles and as a propellant and refrigerant. LPG can be obtained primarily as propane, butane or a mixture of the two. A powerful odorant is added so that it is easily detected.

LPG is flammable and heavier than air so that it will settle, and may accumulate, in low spots such as drains and basements. Here it could present a fire, explosion or suffocation hazard.

Revision exercise

Identify classes for fire, with an example of the type of fuel. (8)

Exam tip

Look up further information that can be found about properties and safe storage of liquefied petroleum gas (LPG) at:

http://www.hse.gov.uk/gas/lpg/
http://www.hse.gov.uk/gas/lpg/about.htm.

Describe the principles of fire growth and fire spread

Key revision points

▶ Factors that influence fire growth rates and smoke movement
▶ Methods of heat transfer: conduction, convection, radiation and direct burning and how they contribute to fire and smoke spread through buildings and to neighbouring properties
▶ The development of a fire under free burning conditions and a fire in enclosed conditions
▶ The conditions in which flashover and backdraught (backdraft) may occur

Factors that influence fire growth rates and smoke movement

- ▶ building design:
  - ▷ cavities
  - ▷ ducts
  - ▷ shafts
- ▶ insulated core panels;
- ▶ construction materials:
  - ▷ timber
  - ▷ bricks
  - ▷ concrete
  - ▷ metal
  - ▷ building boards/slabs
- ▶ internal linings;
- ▶ ventilation levels; and
- ▶ contents of the premises.

Principles of heat transmission and fire spread

Direct burning

Is when the flames/heat reach the combustible materials and ignite them.

Conduction

Is the transfer of heat through solid materials involving the molecule-to-molecule transfer of heat through conducting solids such as metal beams or pipes to other parts of the building and igniting combustible or flammable materials.

Convection

Is the transfer of heat from a liquid or gas (i.e. air, flames or fire products) to a solid or liquid surface. Heat can be carried by rising air currents (convection) to cause a build-up of hot gases.

123

Radiation

Involves the emission of heat in the form of infrared radiation, which can raise temperatures of adjacent materials – for example, electric fire elements.

A fire in an enclosed room is however a totally different phenomena to an open burning fire. The speed of fire growth can be devastating, with two fire phenomena of specific note: **flashover** and **backdraught**.

Flashover

▶ Flashover occurs within a building or structure.
▶ As the fire starts it will grow and develop on an object – for example, furniture. This releases its energy, and it continues to heat up the room.
▶ Hot gases collect near the ceiling.
▶ They start to transfer their energy primarily by radiation down to the burning object.
▶ The burning object absorbs that heat, as do the other objects in the room.
▶ When they reach a point where they are as nearly hot as their ignition temperature they will burst into flames.

Backdraught (Backdraft)

▶ Backdraft is a low-level explosion in building fires.
▶ A fire in a building that is closed (no doors open or windows).
▶ The fire doesn't have enough air to continue to burn.
▶ From a flaming fire, it becomes a smouldering fire, due to lack of oxygen.
▶ It is releasing fuel but no oxygen to react with.
▶ When the building becomes unsealed (from a door or window,) air enters. The air starts to move around that room, and it mixes with the fuel-rich environment caused by the fire.
▶ It finds an ignition source and causes an explosion.

Revision exercise

Describe the principles of the two fire phenomena:

A Flashover (4)
B Backdraught (Backdraft). (4)

Exam tip

When DESCRIBE is used, write your answers so that some-one who is not familiar with the topic would be able to understand what you are writing about.

You can still use sentences, starting a new one on a new line.

Outline the principles of explosion and explosive combustion

Key revision points

▶ Meaning of deflagration and detonation
▶ Common materials involved in explosions
▶ The mechanism of types of explosion, such as gas and vapour explosion (including boiling liquid expanding vapour explosion – BLEVE) and dust explosion (including primary and secondary explosion)
▶ The principles of preventing explosions
▶ The principles for controlling explosions.

Further fire terminology used in fire safety

Deflagration

A process of **subsonic** combustion whereby the flame front propagates through the un-burnt material by thermal conductivity – that is, the burning material heats the next layer of un-burnt material and ignites this and continues through the layer. Hot burning material heats the next layer of cold material until it ignites (e.g. propane, butane).

Detonation

A process of combustion whereby a **supersonic** shock wave propagates through the material and ignites it. Shock wave compresses material in front so that it ignites (e.g. hydrogen, acetylene).

Common materials involved in explosions

▶ flammable liquids;
▶ flammable gases;
▶ flammable vapours;
▶ combustible materials – for example dusts (wood, flour, cotton, custard powder, etc.; and
▶ explosive materials.

Mechanism of types of explosions: Vapour cloud explosion

A vapour cloud explosion may be confined for example in a tank or vessel or unconfined. Its key principles include the presence of flammable vapour at a concentration between the upper and lower explosive limits and an ignition source that exceeds the minimum ignition energy.

Unconfined Vapour Cloud Explosion (UVCE)

▶ May travel a considerable distance before igniting.
▶ Or they may be dispersed to a concentration below the lower explosive limit depending on conditions.

Confined Vapour Cloud Explosion (CVCE)

▶ Vessel or containment rupture may occur resulting in a rapid release of liquefied gas.

▶ Damage to people and property may be caused by the pressure wave and thermal radiation.

Mechanism of types of explosions: Boiling Liquid Expanding Vapour Explosion (BLEVE)

For the BLEVE to occur, the following stages must take place:

▶ Appropriate fuel such as LPG in a vessel.
▶ Presence of an external heat source.
▶ Increase in pressure within the vessel leading to the release of vapour through a relief valve.
▶ Expulsion (and ignition) of vapour via the relief valve.
▶ Rising temperature of the vapour space and vessel walls above the liquid surface.
▶ Development of overpressure/failure of metal in the vessel.
▶ Vessel rupture with the emission of ignited boiling liquid.
▶ Vapour resulting in a fireball producing substantial thermal radiation.
▶ Potential for debris from the vessel to become missiles.

Mechanism of types of explosions: Dust explosion

A dust explosion is an initial (primary) explosion causing dust that has accumulated to be dislodged. This dust, if ignited, causes additional (secondary) explosions, which can result in damage that is more severe than the original explosion due to increased concentrations and quantities of dispersed combustible dust.

Dust explosion pentangle

1 Fuel (combustible dust).
2 Heat/Ignition (flame).
3 Oxygen in air.

127

4 Dispersion of dust particles.

5 Confinement of dust cloud.

For example, see General Foods, Banbury 1981.

http://www.hse.gov.uk/food/dustexplosion.htm.

Inerting, including the advantages and disadvantages of reduced oxygen atmospheres

The partial or complete substitution of the air or flammable atmosphere by an inert gas is a very effective method of explosion prevention. Inerting is normally only considered when the flammable or explosive hazard cannot be eliminated by any other means – i.e. substitution of flammable material with non-flammable adjustment of process conditions to ensure substances are below flammable limits. Gases that can be used for inerting include nitrogen, carbon dioxide, argon, etc.

Principles for controlling explosions

These are:

▶ suppression;
▶ venting:
  ▷ pressure relief valves,
  ▷ bursting discs, and
  ▷ explosion venting panels,
▶ containment; and
▶ cooling.

Revision exercise

State the meaning of:

A BLEVE (2)

B CVCE (2)

C UVCE. (2)

Exam tip

Examples included are for reference purposes only – you will not need to know these for the exam.

Further reading – the following go beyond what is required for this course; however, you may find them interesting.

▶ Buncefield (unconfined vapour cloud explosion) http://www.hse.gov.uk/comah/buncefield/buncefield-report.pdf

▶ Report
Flixborough (unconfined vapour cloud explosion) http://www.hse.gov.uk/comah/sragtech/caseflixboroug74.htm

▶ Mexico City (boiling liquid expanding vapour explosion) http://www.hse.gov.uk/comah/sragtech/casepemex84.htm

▶ Hickson and Welch (confined vapour cloud explosion) http://www.hse.gov.uk/comah/sragtech/casehickwel92.htm

▶ Texas City Refinery, 2005 (explosion) http://www.csb.gov/bp-america-refinery-explosion/

▶ Conocophillips Humber Refinery, 2001 http://www.hse.gov.uk/comah/conocophillips.pdf.

References

1 Available at: http://www.britannica.com/topic-browse/Chemistry/Chemical-Reactions/2

2 British Standards Institute (BSI) (2012) *PAS79: 2012 Fire Risk Assessment: Guidance and a Recommended Methodology*. London: BSI. Available at: http://shop.bsigroup.com/ProductDetail/?pid=000000000030251919

2.3

Causes and prevention of fires and explosions

Explain the causes of fires and explosions in typical work activities ☐

Outline appropriate control measures to minimise fire and explosion risks ☐

Explain the causes of fires and explosions in typical work activities

Key revision points

▶ Common sources of ignition of accidental fires
▶ Sources of fuel
▶ Sources of oxygen
▶ Factors influencing the severity and frequency of an arson attack
▶ Fire and explosion risks from flammable materials in use, storage and transport within the workplace
▶ Concept of fire load
▶ Fire risks in construction and maintenance work.

Common sources of ignition of accidental fires

Fire prevention, which forms a significant part of the fire risk assessment, requires that ignition of combustible materials are controlled within the workplace.

The following are examples of possible ignition sources within the work place:[1]

▶ electrical sources of ignition;
▶ smoking;
▶ arson;
▶ portable heaters and heating installations;
▶ cooking;
▶ lightning;
▶ housekeeping;
▶ hazards introduced by outside contractors and building works;
▶ dangerous substances; and
▶ process fire hazards:

   ▷ hot work (welding, grinding, etc.),
   ▷ overheating of machinery, and
   ▷ spontaneous ignition of oil and solvent soaked materials.

132

The following are examples of possible fuel sources within the work place:

▶ paper and cardboard;
▶ furniture, fixtures and fittings;
▶ structural materials;
▶ wall and ceiling linings;
▶ flammable liquids;
▶ flammable gases (cylinders and piped gas);
▶ flammable vapours;
▶ combustible materials; and
▶ explosive materials.

The following are examples of possible oxygen sources within the work place:

▶ heating and ventilation systems (HAVS);
▶ natural ventilation (open windows);
▶ oxidizing materials; and
▶ oxygen cylinders.

Fire and explosion risks from flammable materials

Increase level of risk from use, storage and transport of flammable materials within the workplace:

▶ lack of training and supervision;
▶ lack of safe system of work;
▶ worker error;
▶ failure of equipment;
▶ unsuitability of equipment;
▶ lack of ventilation;
▶ inadequate storage facilities; and
▶ inadequate transport facilities.

Factors influencing the severity and frequency of an arson attack

Arson is a social problem, a serious crime and also the most common cause of fire. At least one fire in four is deliberately started. Arson causes society extensive material damage and economic losses, and it creates insecurity and suffering for many people. Arson is predominantly a problem associated with young people. Young people are responsible for committing more than 50% of arson fires. In spite of the large number of different measures taken both by national governments and local authorities, it has been difficult to bring about a lasting change in this unfavourable development.[2]

Reasons for starting deliberate fires

▶ profit/insurance fraud;
▶ animosity;
▶ vandalism;
▶ crime concealment;
▶ political objectives;
▶ terrorism; and
▶ psychopathological factors.

Factors influencing the severity and frequency of an arson attack

▶ location;
▶ security; and
▶ access.

Fire and explosion risks from flammable materials in use, storage and transport within the workplace

Small quantities of dangerous goods can be found in most workplaces. Whatever they are used for, the storage and use of such goods can pose a serious hazard unless basic safety principles are followed.

Concept of fire load

▶ In fire engineering literature the quantity of combustibles within an enclosure is termed the 'fire load'.
▶ Fire load represents the total energy that can be released in a compartment as a result of a fire.
▶ Fire loads are determined from surveys.

134

▶ Fire load governs the initial fire growth rate.
▶ Fire load density refers to the quantity of fuel per unit area. It is normally expressed in terms of MJ/m^2 or kg/m^2.
▶ BS 4422 defines fire load as 'quantity of heat which could be released by the complete combustion of all the combustible materials in a volume, including the facings of all bounding surfaces'.
▶ BSEN 1991–1–2:2002 states that the fire load should consist of all combustible building contents and the relevant combustible parts of the construction, including linings and finishings.

Fire risks in construction and maintenance work

▶ Site storage of combustible and flammable materials such as:
  ▷ LPG cylinders and other gases, and
  ▷ drums of fuel.
▶ Waste disposal considerations;
▶ Demolition hazards;
▶ Use of oxy-fuel equipment; and
▶ Temporary electrical installations.

Revision exercise

Identify EIGHT common sources of ignition found in the workplace. (8)

Exam tip

Consider the examples of possible fuel sources, within a (or your) work place and link them to the following headings (from Element 1):
Class A – solids
Class B – liquids
Class C – gasses
Class D – metals
Class F – cooking oils.

Outline appropriate control measures to minimise fire and explosion risks

> ### Key revision points
>
> ▶ Control of sources of ignition
> ▶ Control of sources of fuel
> ▶ Control of sources of oxygen
> ▶ Safe systems of work
> ▶ Actions to minimise risks from arson.

Control of sources of ignition

Factors to consider include:

▶ Intrinsically safe electrical equipment for use in flammable and explosive atmospheres; zoning of hazardous locations/use of mobile phones.
▶ Maintenance and portable appliance testing of portable electrical equipment.
▶ Designated smoking areas, use of fireproof cigarette bins.
▶ Shielding to block radiant heat and sparks.
▶ Maintain separation of ignition sources and fuel sources.
▶ Effective static control systems:

  ▷ Bonding or earthing continuity between pieces of equipment particularly portable equipment such as containers for carrying highly flammable substances, piping, filling funnels, drip trays, and the like.
  ▷ Not wearing outer clothing that generates static charges. In practice this usually means avoiding human-made fibres and using cotton only.
  ▷ Using conductive footwear to leak static charges to ground (these must not be used by electricians as they conduct electricity and will not protect them against electric shock).
  ▷ Avoiding free fall of highly flammable liquids from one container to another unless anti-static additives have been

136

put into the liquid or its natural properties will not hold static charges. Filling funnels should reach down to as near to the bottom of the container being filled as possible.

Control of sources of fuel

Factors to consider include:

▶ Safe storage, transport and use of flammable, highly flammable and combustible materials.
▶ Design and installation of storage facilities.
▶ Inspection and maintenance programmes, safe waste disposal methods.
▶ Housekeeping.
▶ Control of fire load.

Safe storage and use of flammable liquids

This can be accomplished by addressing the following five areas:

V entilation

I gnition

C ontainment

E xchange

S eparation.[3]

Ventilation

Is there plenty of fresh air where flammable liquids or gases are stored and used? Good ventilation will mean that any vapours given off from a spill, leak or release from any process, will be rapidly dispersed.

Ignition

Have all the obvious ignition sources been removed from storage and handling areas? Ignition sources can be varied and they include sparks from electrical equipment or welding and cutting tools, hot surfaces, open flames from heating equipment, smoking materials, etc.

Containment

Are your flammable substances kept in suitable containers? If you have a spill, will it be contained and prevented from spreading to other parts of the working area? Use of lidded containers and spillage catchment trays, for example, can help to prevent spillages spreading.

Exchange

Can you exchange a flammable substance for a less flammable one? Can you eliminate flammable substances from the process altogether? You may be able to think of other ways of carrying out the job more safely.

Separation

Are flammable substances stored and used well away from other processes and general storage areas? Can they be separated by a physical barrier, wall or partition? Separating your hazards in this manner will contribute to a safer workplace.

Principles of preventing explosions

Principles of preventing explosions can be achieved by ensuring there is:

▶ good housekeeping;
▶ good ventilation;
▶ safe storage;
▶ safe handling of explosive materials;
▶ control of detonation sources;
▶ cooling; and
▶ inerting.

Examiner's tip

This is an example of an identify answer – providing a list.

Storing and handling flammable solvents

Precautions that should be considered when storing and handling flammable solvents in small containers include:

▶ Controlling the disposal of flammable waste and providing suitable appliances for fighting fire.
▶ Ensuring that empty containers are tightly closed and stored outside the building or in a store constructed of fire resisting materials.
▶ Labelling the containers clearly with information about their contents.
▶ Limiting the quantities stored and the amounts in use.
▶ Marking the storage area in which they are held.
▶ Removing likely sources of ignition.
▶ Selecting containers that are suitable for the purpose.
▶ Taking measures to prevent vapour build-up by the provision of a good standard of ventilation and to prevent or reduce the impact of spillages by using non-spill caps or bunding the area where the containers are held.

Examiner's tip

This is an example of an outline answer – providing short sentences.

Control of sources of oxygen

Factors to consider include:

▶ closing doors and windows;
▶ shutting off ventilation/air conditioning systems/ducting; and
▶ safe use and storage of oxidizing materials.

Additional factors to reduce the risk of a fire

▶ Control of smoking and smoking materials.
▶ Controlling hot work by permits or by creation of designated areas.

▶ Ensuring that electrical systems are not overloaded.

▶ Ensuring ventilation outlets on equipment are not obstructed.

▶ Good housekeeping to prevent accumulation of waste paper and other combustible materials.

▶ Isolating equipment that is not in use.

▶ Providing proper storage facilities for flammable liquids away from sources of ignition.

▶ Regular inspection of electrical equipment for damage.

▶ Regular lubrication of machinery to prevent sparks.

▶ Segregating incompatible chemicals and implementing security procedures to reduce risk of arson.

Safe systems of work – for example, *when undertaking oxyacetylene welding in a workplace*

▶ Closing cylinders at the valve when not in use.

▶ Completing user checks of the equipment before starting the operation.

▶ Ensuring the gas cylinders are not heated by the flame or by stray arcs from adjacent electrical equipment.

▶ Fitting the torch unit with non-return valves and flash back arrestors to the outlet of the regulators.

▶ Making use of a permit to work system. ∙

▶ Minimising the amount of combustible material in the area of the welding operation.

▶ Providing fire fighting equipment and maintaining a fire watch.

▶ Storing oxygen and acetylene cylinders in an upright position in a well-ventilated area and away from sources of heat and sparks.

▶ Using crimped hose connections and not jubilee clips.

▶ Using hoses that are as short as possible and are colour-coded – red for acetylene and blue for oxygen.

▶ Using regulators (gas cylinder heads) to the appropriate standard.

▶ Using trained and competent staff to carry out the welding operation.

Actions to minimise risks from arson[4]

▶ Closed containers for combustible materials are not kept nearer than four metres from the building.

▶ External lighting is not damaged.

▶ Heaps of combustible materials, leaves and dry twigs in corners or similar, that are not easily overlooked, are removed.

▶ Loading bays are cleared of combustible material and anything else that should not be there.

▶ Open containers for combustible materials are not kept nearer than 6 metres from the building.

▶ Refuse or empty packaging or other combustible material is not stored along the facade or under a canopy.

▶ Refuse storage rooms, stores, etc. are locked.

▶ There are no ladders or other material that can be used to climb up to the roof.

▶ Ensure windows and roof lights are closed.

Revision exercise

Identify FIVE key considerations for safe storage and use of flammable liquids. (5)

Exam tip

When considering control measures – make sure you include the obvious answers too!

References

1 British Standards Institute (BSI) (2012) *PAS79: 2012 Fire Risk Assessment: Guidance and a Recommended Methodology*. London: BSI. Available at: http://shop.bsigroup.com/ProductDetail/?pid=000000000030251919

2 Available at: http://www.cfpa-e.eu/wp-content/uploads/files/guidelines/Guideline_No_8_2004.pdf

3 Available at: http://www.hse.gov.uk/PUBNS/indg227.pdf

4 Available at: http://www.cfpa-e.eu/wp-content/uploads/files/guidelines/CFPA_E_Guideline_No_16_2008.pdf

2.4

Fire protection in buildings

Learning outcomes

Outline the means of fire protection and prevention of fire and smoke spread within buildings in relation to building construction and design ☐

Explain the requirements of a means of escape ☐

Outline the methods and systems available to give early warning in case of fire, both for life safety and for property protection ☐

Outline the selection procedures for basic fire extinguishing methods for both life risk and for process risk ☐

Explain the requirements for ensuring access for the fire service is provided and maintained ☐

Outline steps to minimise the environmental impact of fire and fire fighting operations ☐

Outline the means of fire protection and prevention of fire and smoke spread within buildings in relation to building construction and design

Key revision points

▶ The role of the Building Regulations 2010
▶ Elements of structure according to the Building Regulations 'Approved Document B'
▶ Properties and requirements of fire resistance for elements of structure
▶ Compartmentation to inhibit spread of fire and smoke within buildings
▶ Fire-resisting dampers (mechanical or intumescent)
▶ Internal fire growth
▶ Fire resisting walls
▶ Alarm systems linked to forced ventilation systems
▶ Means of preventing external fire spread.

Role of building regulations 2010

The implementation of Building Regulations is a historic precedent and can be traced back to the Great Fire of London in 1666, following which Charles II decreed that walls between buildings (party walls) must be constructed of brick or stone, and that buildings with timber claddings must be far enough apart to prevent the spread of fire from one to another. Building and fire safety legislation was reactive in its origin, starting with one piece of legislation with regards to both buildings and fire safety: the London Buildings Act 1667.

The current Building Regulations 2010 plays a key part in fire safety with regards to the design of buildings.

Building work must be carried out so that it complies with the applicable requirements set out in Building Regulations 2010, Parts

A to P of Schedule 1. The requirements in Schedule 1 relate to structural safety (Part A), fire safety (Part B), etc.[1]

Building regulations 2010, schedule 1 requirements[2]

Part A Structure

A1 Loading
The building shall be constructed so that the combined dead, imposed and wind loads are sustained and transmitted by it to the ground

A2 Ground movement
The building shall be constructed so that ground movement will not impair the stability of any part of the building

A3 Disproportionate collapse
The building shall be constructed so that in the event of an accident the building will not suffer collapse to an extent disproportionate to the cause

Elements of structure

Elements of structure is the term applied to the main structural load bearing elements:

▶ frames;
▶ floors; and
▶ load bearing walls.

Fire resistance for elements

Fire resistance for elements include:

▶ Resistance to collapse.
▶ Fire and smoke penetration and transfer of excessive heat.
▶ Resistance of fire doors and glazing.
▶ Significance of any immediately visible damage and the need to repair it.

Principles of fire protection in buildings

Factors to take into account include:

▶ Surface spread:
  ▷ Class 0 – Materials suitable for circulation spaces and escape routes
  ▷ Class 1 – Surface of very low flame spread
  ▷ Class 2 – Surface of low flame spread
  ▷ Class 3 – Surface of medium flame spread
  ▷ Class 4 – Surface of rapid flame spread
▶ Fire resistance of structural elements
▶ Insulating materials
▶ Fire compartmentation.

Compartmentation to inhibit spread of fire and smoke within buildings

Compartmentation in buildings serves a number of purposes:

▶ Providing a physical barrier for fire and confining it to its zone of origin for a specified time.
▶ Reducing the number of employees immediately at risk and the travel distance of those who need to escape to a place of relative safety.
▶ Reducing the extent of the spread of smoke, heat and toxic gases and minimising the risk of them entering protected escape routes.
▶ Enabling phased evacuations and offering the possibility of providing safe havens for vulnerable persons.

Ways of achieving an adequate level of compartmentation within a building include:

▶ Dividing it into discrete fire resisting zones.
▶ Using fire-resisting elements such as brick walls for the structure.
▶ Protecting structural materials such as concrete and steel.
▶ Providing fire protection for floors – for example, by the use of low density concrete.
▶ Fitting fire resisting doors and fire resistant glazing.

146

▶ Sealing voids and enclosing lifts by compartment walls.
▶ Arranging for the compartmentation of roof voids – for example, by the use of fabric cavity-barriers.
▶ Fitting fire dampers in duct work and fire stopping where services pass through compartments.

Fire-resisting dampers: Mechanical or intumescent

Fire and/or smoke resisting dampers are used to prevent fire and/or smoke moving through heating, ventilation and air conditioning (HVAC) systems.[3]

▶ **Mechanical dampers** use a motorised system, which is linked to smoke sensors; if smoke is detected, then the fire-resistant board or steel shutters (similar to blinds on a window) will close.
▶ **Intumescent dampers** incorporate components, which expand when heated, to halt the passage of fire and/or smoke.

Internal fire growth

Factors that affect internal fire growth:

▶ wall lining materials (including over-painting);
▶ fixtures;
▶ fittings; and
▶ contents.

Growth Rate	Typical real fires
Slow	▶ Densely packed wood products
Medium	▶ Solid wood furniture (desks)
	▶ Individual furniture items with small amounts of plastic
Fast	▶ High stacked wood pallets
	▶ Cartons on pallets
	▶ Some upholstered furniture
Ultra Fast	▶ Upholstered furniture
	▶ High stacked plastic materials
	▶ Thin wood furniture (wardrobes)

Fire resisting walls

Wall coverings that are fire resistant include:

▶ asbestos cement;
▶ brick;
▶ calcium silicate boards;
▶ concrete;
▶ cement render;
▶ fire-retardant treated wood;
▶ gypsum boards;
▶ insulated core panels/sandwich panels;
▶ rock wool; and
▶ surface lining materials (see following).

Surface lining materials

Properties of surface lining materials that might increase the risk of fire spread and its growth:

▶ Surface lining materials ignitability.
▶ Rates of surface flame spread and heat release.
▶ Amount of smoke produced when ignited.
▶ Propensity for producing flaming droplets.

Examples of surface lining materials that could be used to reduce the risk of fire spread and its growth:

▶ exposed brickwork;
▶ exposed blockwork;
▶ mineral fibre board;
▶ wood wool slabs;
▶ plaster board and skim;
▶ intumescent linings;
▶ fire resistant glass;
▶ concrete; and
▶ stone/ceramic tiles.

Materials with a resistance to ignition and with low rates of surface flame spread and heat release would help to limit the spread of fire, the production of smoke and the rate of fire growth and would maximise the time available for escape routes to be used safely.

Alarm systems linked to forced ventilation systems

Forced ventilation system installed in a building includes fans, ventilation pumps, pressurisation systems, inlets and outlets of ventilation. Smoke extraction systems serve to prevent smoke spreading to some critical areas, reduce the smoke temperature and improve visibility by taking action such as diluting the smoke with fresh air.[4]

Means of preventing external fire spread

Factors to consider for the means of preventing external fire spread include:

▶ construction of external walls and roofs;
▶ distance between buildings;
▶ use/activities undertaken at premises;
▶ surrounding premises; and
▶ the role of external walls in protecting escape routes at the boundaries.

Revision exercise

Identify the **FOUR fire** growth rates and **state** an example of real fires. (8)

Exam tip

When considering fire growth rates – look at your workplace and try to estimate the growth rates in different areas/rooms.

Explain the requirements of a means of escape

Key revision points

▶ Understanding of a means of escape
▶ Principles, features and general requirements of means of escape
▶ Management actions to maintain means of escape
▶ Requirements for means of escape for vulnerable people and people with disabilities and/or mobility problems.

Understanding of a means of escape

Floors and ceilings forming escape routes need to maintain fire resistance. Other factors to be considered are:

▶ The number of occupants to be evacuated.
▶ The number of fire escape routes.
▶ The length of time it will take for all occupants to escape to a place of safety and whether this time is reasonable.
▶ Whether all escape routes are easily identifiable, unobstructed and adequately illuminated.
▶ Whether the type and size of exits are suitable and sufficient for the number and type of persons who will use them taking into account the presence of disabled personnel.
▶ The protection of the escape routes including staircases.
▶ The adequacy of the arrangements for persons with disabilities.

Available Safe Egress Time (ASET)

Is the amount of time that elapses between fire ignition and the development of untenable conditions.

Required Safe Egress Time (RSET)

Is the amount of time (also measured from fire ignition) that is required for occupants to evacuate a building or space and reach the building exterior or a protected exit enclosure.

150

Table 1 Principles, features and general requirements of means of escape

Available Safe Egress Time (ASET)					
Required Safe Egress Time (RSET)					**Safety Margin**
Detection Time	Alarm Time	Recognition Time	Response Time	Travel Time	
Ignition	Detection				Evacuation

The following principles, features and general requirements of means of escape include:

▶ Providing alternative escape routes.
▶ Understanding that all persons within the premises should be able to reach a place of ultimate safety before life-threatening conditions arise; either unaided or with the assistance of staff but without fire rescue service assistance:
  ▷ Required Safe Egress Time (RSET), and
  ▷ Available Safe Egress Time (ASET).
▶ Maximum travel distances (escape distances).
▶ Number and size of escape routes for number of occupants.
▶ Requirements for escape stairs, passageways and doors.
▶ Use of door releases and other escape devices (including the need for these to be fail safe).
▶ Protection of escape routes.
▶ Emergency escape lighting (EEL) – common forms, modes of operation and signage; siting of luminaires and 'Point of Emphasis'; limitations of emergency generators.
▶ Design for progressive horizontal evacuation.
▶ Final exit to a place of safety, etc.
▶ Use of door releases and other escape devices (including the need for these to be fail safe).

Management actions to maintain means of escape

The following are management actions to maintain means of escape:

▶ Regular checking of means of escape for:
  ▷ blocked exits;
  ▷ faulty emergency lighting;
  ▷ faulty fire doors; and
  ▷ fire doors propped open, incorrectly.
▶ Recording findings in fire logbook.

Guidance to travel distances is outlined in the DCLG guides – for example, for offices and shops, in normal risk premises:

Where more than one escape route is provided   45 m travel distance.
Where only a single escape route is provided   18 m travel distance.

The actual distance is measured to:

▶ a protected stairway enclosure (a storey exit);
▶ a separate fire compartment from which there is a final exit to a place of total safety; or
▶ the nearest available final exit.

An emergency escape lighting system should normally cover the following:

▶ each exit door;
▶ escape routes;
▶ intersections of corridors;
▶ outside each final exit and on external escape routes;
▶ emergency escape signs;
▶ stairways so that each flight receives adequate light;
▶ changes in floor level;
▶ windowless rooms and toilet accommodation exceeding 8m^2;
▶ fire fighting equipment;
▶ fire alarm call points;
▶ equipment that would need to be shut down in an emergency;
▶ lifts; and
▶ areas in premises greater than 60m^2.

Providing a means of escape in a workplace so that all employees are able to reach a place of safety in the event of a fire could be accomplished by:

▶ Ensuring there is sufficient number of exit routes required – with regard to the size of the premises and number of people within.

▶ Ensuring there is sufficient width to the exit routes – to cater for wheel chairs and the number of people within.

▶ Final exit door should open quickly and easily and preferably outwards.

▶ Fire exit routes should be protected with fire resistant materials and the fitting of self-closing fire doors along corridors and protected routes, where required.

▶ The introduction of procedures for disabled persons including the provision of safe havens and fire fighting lifts.

▶ The location of fire fighting equipment along exit routes.

▶ The means for raising the alarm that should have sufficient call points and be audible throughout the premises.

▶ The need to appoint responsible persons such as fire marshals and emergency services liaison personnel.

▶ The provision of adequate signage for, and emergency lighting, along exit routes.

▶ Travel distances should comply within suitable guidelines involved depending on the fire risk and the number of exits.

Fire doors

Fire doors are provided in buildings to protect escape routes from the effects of fire so that occupants can safely reach the final exit and also to protect the contents and/or the structure of the building by limiting the spread of fire and smoke. Fire doors provided to protect the means of escape should:

▶ Be capable of achieving a minimum fire resistance (FR) for integrity of 30 minutes.

▶ Be easy to open and not locked, obstructed or offer any resistance.

▶ Be fitted with intumescent strips and seals.

▶ Be self-closing to prevent spread of fire and smoke.

▶ Be wide enough for the number of people likely to use them.

▶ Lead to a place of safety.

▶ Not be wedged open (unless with fire standard approved automatic door stop which releases the door upon activation of the fire alarm system).

▶ Open in the direction of travel (unless a fire risk assessment deems this acceptable due to low number of occupants).

Requirements for means of escape for vulnerable people and people with disabilities and/or mobility problems

▶ Use of evacuation lifts and refuges areas, prior to evacuating before fire authority arrives.

▶ Use of visual (including graphics), aural and tactile way-finding and exit sign systems

▶ Development of Personal Emergency Evacuation Plans (PEEPs).

Revision exercise

Describe the meaning of ASET and RSET. (4)

Identify surface lining materials that could be used to reduce the risk of fire spread and its growth. (4)

Exam tip

Some questions will be set from more than one learning outcome.

Outline the methods and systems available to give early warning in case of fire, both for life safety and property protection

Key revision points

▶ Fire alarm and fire detection systems
▶ Types of automatic fire detection, their limitations and links with other systems and equipment – e.g. fire doors and fire extinguishing systems
▶ Categories of fire alarm and detection systems and their objectives (BS 5839, Part 1 and Part 6)
▶ Fire alarm zoning, the need for zone plans and their value to the FRS Alarm signalling, common alarm devices and their limitations
▶ Emergency Voice Communication (EVC) Systems
▶ Use of alarm receiving centres
▶ Manual and automatic systems
▶ Factors to be considered in the selection of fire detection and fire alarm systems
▶ Requirements for certification, maintenance and testing of fire detection and alarm systems.

Fire alarm and fire detection systems

The reasons for installing an automatic fire detection system:

▶ Detection of a fire at an early stage together with an indication of the location of its source.
▶ The protection it provides for specific areas such as sleeping areas, kitchens and boiler rooms.
▶ Its operation without human intervention providing early warning to the occupants of a building of the existence of a fire and thus enabling a controlled evacuation at an early stage.
▶ Its ability to obtain a rapid response from the fire service that might consequently result in damage limitation.

155

Types of automatic fire detection[5]

Optical smoke detectors
Are activated when smoke enters the chamber of the detector, light is scattered on to the photo-diode.

Ionisation smoke detectors
Are activated when smoke enters one of the two chambers of the detector. This causes an increase of voltage at the point where the inner and outer chambers join, due to the irradiated air.

Heat detectors
Are activated when thermistor reaches a specified rate (standard devices report an alarm at 55°C). Thermistors have a resistance that rapidly decreases with an increase in temperature.

Beam Detectors
Are activated when there is a break of the beam of infrared light from the transmitter to the receiver.

Manual Call Points (break glass points)
Are activated when the break glass is pressed.

Alarms can be audio (aural), visual or vibration

▶ Audio alarms:
  ▷ sounders/beacons;
  ▷ emergency voice communication (EVC) systems;
  ▷ rotary bell;
  ▷ horn/whistle;
  ▷ being verbally informed 'Fire!'; and
  ▷ radios/pagers.
▶ Visual alarms:
  ▷ flashing beacons/lights.
▶ Vibration alarms:
  ▷ pagers/trembler alarms (can be used for those working in noisy work areas and for hearing impaired workers).

156

Table 2 Categories of fire alarm and detection systems and their objectives (as per BS 5839, Part 1 and Part 6)

Type	Coverage
Manual system:	
Category M:	Manual all points emergency exits.
Life risk/protection: In this situation the objective is to protect people from loss of life or injury:	
Category L1:	Total coverage
Category L2:	Escape routes, rooms adjacent to emergency routes and high-risk areas (L2 = L3 + L5)
Category L3:	Escape routes and rooms adjacent to emergency routes
Category L4:	Escape routes
Category L5:	High-risk areas
Property risk/protection: In this situation the objective is to summon the Fire and Rescue Service in the early stages of a fire:	
Category P1:	Total coverage
Category P2:	High-risk areas

Circumstances where automatic fire detection might be appropriate include:

▶ Areas where a fire could start undetected such as a storeroom or an unmanned building or where lone working is carried out.

▶ In areas where vulnerable people are present or in areas providing sleeping accommodation and where it will assist in the rapid initiation of phased evacuations.

▶ Where it might provide a compensating feature for inadequate structural fire protection or where there is limited means of escape such as in inner rooms or dead ends.

▶ Where rapid fire detection is required such as in areas where flammable materials are stored.

▶ Where smoke control or ventilation is controlled by automatic detection systems.

Fire alarm zoning, the need for zone plans and their value to the FRS Alarm signalling, common alarm devices and their limitations

Fire Alarm Zone Diagram/Plan should comply with BS 5839. A Zone Diagram/Plan is an installed topographic drawing of the protected premises indicating the fire alarm zone system with clearly identifiable colour-coded areas. This will assist the fire service in locating the fire. Zoned fire alarm system provides a quick means of identifying where a fire has started, enables a swift location of the fire by the Fire Authority and assists in the structured staged evacuation of the building.

Emergency Voice Communication (EVC) Systems

Emergency Voice Communication System is the term used for both 'Fire Fighting Telephone Systems' and 'Disabled Refuge Communication Systems'.

The EVC systems purpose is to assist the orderly evacuation of disabled or mobility-impaired people and to enhance fire fighters communication during emergencies.

Use of alarm receiving centres

Both automatic and manual fire detection systems can be connected to an alarm-receiving centre. This connection is normally via a telephone line. The use of such a monitoring system can provide significant benefits:

▶ Alarm receiving centres normally provide the facility to contact the emergency services.
▶ A system provides constant monitoring of the fire detection system: constant meaning 24 hours, seven days a week.
▶ The majority of fires start after normal working hours, and a long period of time could elapse before the fire is detected if the building is unoccupied, and not linked to an alarm-receiving centre.
▶ There could be a situation in which the person nominated to call the fire and emergency services is unavailable.

158

▶ Having an alarm-receiving centre monitoring a premises may reduce the insurance premium or be a requirement to get insurance in the first place.

Manual and automatic systems

Component parts of a fire alarm system are:

▶ **Automatic fire detection** such as a heat or smoke detector which allows for the automatic detection of a fire and the activation of the alarm without human intervention.
▶ **Alarm sounders** that provide an audible warning of the activation of a fire alarm.
▶ **Flashing beacons** or **trembler alarms** which provide visual warning of the activation of the alarm.
▶ **Fire panel** that provides information to the fire service of the location of the activation of the alarm.
▶ **Alarm zones** where premises are divided into zones to enable a quicker location of the position of the fire to be made and to allow for staged evacuation from the premises.
▶ **Manual call points** to enable manual operation of the fire alarm by worker.

Factors to be considered in the selection of fire detection and fire alarm systems include

▶ Life risk (of those within the premises).
▶ Non-life risk factors: premises, process, products.
▶ Requirements for vulnerable people and people with disabilities and/or mobility problems.
▶ Social behaviour and minimising false alarms including the behavioural issues of those in the premises.

Human behaviour – in response to an alarm

The following are possible responses to a fire alarm:

▶ Ignore the alarm:
  ▷ Did not recognise it; or
  ▷ Believed it to be a false alarm.

159

▶ Out of curiosity attempted to investigate what was happening.
▶ Theft / dishonest gain during alarm.
▶ Comply with procedures and use the designated fire escape routes; await instructions.
▶ Delay evacuation to collect their belongings.
▶ Panic and freeze.

Reducing false alarms from automatic fire detection systems

▶ Installing the appropriate system in all areas – for example, avoiding the use of smoke detectors in kitchens.
▶ Introducing procedures for the regular testing and maintenance of detection systems to avoid malfunction and isolating detectors whilst the maintenance work is being carried out.
▶ Investigating all false alarms to identify the reasons for the alarm and to implement remedial action.
▶ Providing protection on manual call points where they may be set off accidentally such as in store areas where they can be triggered when moving stock.

Requirements for certification, maintenance and testing of fire detection and alarm systems

▶ Local regulations/orders
▶ BS standards/international standards
▶ Manufacturers guidelines
▶ Fire detection and fire warning systems including self-contained smoke detectors and manually operated devices may require testing:
▶ Weekly
  ▷ Check all systems for state of repair and operation. Repair or replace defective units. Test operation of systems, self-contained alarms and manually operated devices.
▶ Annually
  ▷ Full check and test of system by competent service engineer. Clean self-contained smoke alarms and change batteries.

Revision exercise

Identify different categories of fire alarm systems and **state** the type of coverage for the category. **(8)**

Exam tip

Consider the fire alarm system at your place of work – how does it work?

Outline the selection procedures for basic fire extinguishing methods for both life risk and process risk

Key revision points

▶ Factors in the provision, design and application of portable fire-fighting equipment and fixed installations
▶ Extinguishing media
▶ Portable fire fighting equipment
▶ Fixed installations

Factors in the provision, design and application of portable fire-fighting equipment and fixed installations

The following factors should be considered for the provision, design and application of portable fire-fighting equipment and fixed installations:

▶ Local regulations/orders;
▶ BS standards/international standards;
▶ Manufacturer's guidelines;

161

▶ Type and use of premises; and
▶ Company policy with regards to the use of fighting equipment:
  ▷ Operation and safe use for fighting equipment by trained employees, or
  ▷ Fighting equipment is for decoration; do not attempt to tackle the fire.

Portable fire fighting equipment: Siting

Extinguishers should normally be sited:

▶ In prominent positions on brackets or stands.
▶ On escape routes and in similar locations on all floors.
▶ Near room exits, corridors, stairways, landings and lobbies.

The following factors should be considered when siting fire extinguishers:

▶ Extinguishers should be on an escape route.
▶ Elevated to a height so that the carrying handle is 1m from the floor for heavier units and 1.5m for smaller units.
▶ Adjacent to the risk but not too close to prevent use in the event of fire occurring.
▶ Near a door, inside or outside according to occupancy.
▶ In multi-storey buildings at the same position on each storey.
▶ In groups forming 'fire points'.
▶ In shallow recesses where possible.
▶ Away from extremes of temperature within extinguisher temperature ranges.
▶ Maximum 30m travelling distance from a fire to an extinguisher.

Class type / extinguisher type

A – solids	–	Water, Foam, Dry Powder
B – liquids	–	Foam, Dry Powder
C – gases	–	Dry Powder, CO_2
D – metals	–	Specialist Dry Powder
F – cooking oil	–	Wet Chemical
Electrical fires	–	Dry Powder, CO_2

Types of portable fire fighting equipment[6]

Water extinguishers (red)

This type of extinguisher can only be used on Class A fires. They allow the user to direct water onto a fire from a considerable distance. A nine-litre water extinguisher can be quite heavy, and some water extinguishers with additives can achieve the same rating, although they are smaller and therefore considerably lighter. This type of extinguisher is not suitable for use on live electrical equipment.

Foam extinguishers (cream)

This type of extinguisher can be used on Class A or B fires and is particularly suited to extinguishing liquid fires such as petrol and diesel. They should not be used on free-flowing liquid fires unless the operator has been specially trained, as these have the potential to rapidly spread the fire to adjacent material. This type of extinguisher is not suitable for deep-fat fryers or chip pans.

Powder extinguishers (blue)

This type of extinguisher can be used on most classes of fire and achieve a good 'knock down' of the fire. They can be used on fires involving electrical equipment but will almost certainly render that equipment useless. Because they do not cool the fire appreciably, it can re-ignite. Powder extinguishers can create a loss of visibility and may affect people who have breathing problems, and they are not generally suitable for enclosed spaces.

Carbon dioxide extinguishers (black)

This type of extinguisher is particularly suitable for fires involving electrical equipment, as they will extinguish a fire without causing any further damage (except in the case of some electronic equipment – e.g. computers). As with all fires involving electrical equipment, the power should be disconnected if possible.

163

Class 'F' extinguishers

This type of extinguisher is particularly suitable for commercial catering establishments with deep-fat fryers.

Class A fire calculation

Class A – Fires involving solid materials, usually of an organic nature in which combustion normally takes place with the formation of glowing embers.

Minimum quantities of Class A extinguishers required:

Class A materials are generally present in all premises and occupancies. The minimum quantity of extinguishers with an A rating should be calculated as follows:

(a) For any storey with a floor area less than or equal to 400 m^2, there should be:

(1) at least two (2) extinguishers with a class A rating; having

(2) a combined minimum total fire rating of 26A;

(b) For any storey with a floor area exceeding 400 m^2, there should be:

(1) at least two (2) extinguishers with a class A rating; having

(2) a combined minimum total fire rating of 0.065 × floor area of the storey (in square metres).

There should be a minimum of two extinguishers per floor, unless the upper floor area is very small (i.e. below 100m^2) and in single occupancy, in which case, only one extinguisher is required on the upper floor.[7] Small premises, having one or two portable extinguishers of the appropriate type, readily available for use, may be all that is necessary.

Portable fire fighting equipment

Inspections of portable fire fighting equipment are undertaken to ensure that they:

▶ are located in the designated place;
▶ are unobstructed and visible, and that the operating instructions face outwards;

▶ have operating instructions that are clean and legible;
▶ are not obviously damaged;
▶ have a reading in the operable range or position of any pressure gauge or indicator fitted; and
▶ have seals and tamper indicators that are not broken or missing.

Extinguishing media

There are **FOUR** modes of action for fighting a fire. These are:

▶ **Cooling**
  ▷ To reduce the ignition temperature by taking heat out of the fire – using water to limit or reduce the temperature.

▶ **Smothering**
  ▷ Will limit oxygen available and prevent mixture of oxygen and flammable vapour by the use of a foam extinguisher or a fire blanket.

▶ **Starving**
  ▷ Will limit fuel supply – by removing the source of fuel, isolating the flow of flammable liquids or removing wood and textiles, etc.

▶ **Chemical reaction**
  ▷ By interrupting the chain of combustion and combining the hydrogen atoms with chlorine atoms in the hydrocarbon chain.

Fixed installations

These are fire-fighting systems that are normally installed within the structure of the building.

▶ **Hose reels**
  Permanent hose reels provide an effective fire fighting facility. They may offer an alternative, or be in addition to, portable fire fighting equipment. A concern is that untrained people will stay and fight a fire when escape is the safest option.

▶ **Smoke control systems**
  These are complex systems that are provided for life safety of occupants, assistance to fire-fighters and property protection by clearing hot smoke and gases from the building.

▶ **Suppression systems**

Fire suppression systems can include sprinklers and other types of fixed installations designed to automatically operate and suppress a fire.

▷ Sprinkler systems can be very effective in controlling fires. They can be designed to protect life and/or property and may be regarded as a cost-effective solution for reducing the risks created by fire. Where installed, a sprinkler system is usually part of a package of fire precautions in a building and may form an integral part of the fire strategy for the building.

Factors to consider with sprinkler systems include:

▶ Provision of an adequate sprinkler system would be the capacity of water required.
▶ Existence of an adequate and assured water supply.
▶ Availability of an alternative if this was to fail for any reason.
▶ Pumping system would also be important with a diesel back up if the decision was taken to install electrically operated pumps.
▶ Means of activating the system (frangible bulbs or detector activated).
▶ Linkage of the system to alarms.
▶ Spray pattern required.
▶ Area to be covered and the presence of other combustibles.
▶ Height of the storage racks and their distance from the sprinkler heads.
▶ Provision of fire stopping for sprinklers passing through compartmentalisation.
▶ Provision of fire-water run-off and the arrangements to be put in place for testing the equipment.

Revision exercise

Describe the **FOUR** modes of action for fighting a fire. (8)

Exam tip

Consider the types of fire fighting equipment within your workplace – do you have suitable and sufficient coverage?

Explain the requirements for ensuring access for the fire service is provided and maintained

---

Key revision points

▶ Need for vehicle and building access, fire mains/water source and smoke/heat venting of basements
▶ Fire fighting shafts and stairwells
▶ Liaison with fire authority on arrival
▶ Contents of building.

Need for vehicle and building access, fire mains/water source and smoke/heat venting of basements

There should be vehicle and building access for the fire brigade:[8]

▶ There should be vehicle access for a pump appliance to small buildings (those of up to 2,000m^2 with a top storey less than 11m above ground level) to either:
  ▷ 15% of the perimeter; and
  ▷ within 45m of every point on the projected plan area (or 'footprint') of the building.
▶ In the case of a building fitted with fire mains, there should be access for a pumping appliance to within 18m of each fire main inlet connection point.

There should be access to fire mains/water source:

▶ In the UK multi-storey buildings, over 18m high, have to be constructed with fire fighting shafts provided with fire mains.

167

Smoke control system to be provided for any basement storey that has:[9]

▶ A floor area of more than 200m^2
▶ A floor more than 3m below the adjacent ground level
▶ All basement car parks, regardless of the size.

This can be through:

▶ Natural Ventilation; or
▶ Mechanical Ventilation.

Fire fighting shafts and stairways

Fire fighting shafts are provided in larger buildings to help fire-fighters reach floors further away from the building's access point. They are required if there is a floor level 18m or more above fire service access level or a basement more than 10m below.

They enable fire fighting operations to start quickly and in comparative safety by providing a safe route from the point of entry to the floor where the fire has occurred. A fire fighting shaft contains: a protected stairway and lobby – there may be a fire fighting lift. The stairway and lobby require smoke ventilation to allow fire-fighters safe access to every level. The ventilation system is intended to keep the stairway free of smoke and improve conditions in the lobby.

Liaison with fire authority on arrival

This will include:

▶ Providing a point of contact – for example, a fire warden;
▶ Ensuring everyone is out of building; and
▶ Providing location and details of dangerous substances within the premises and surrounding area.

Contents of building

The fire service needs to be aware of the contents of the premises they are attending and provided with details of combustible materials and the substances within the premises.

The fire load of a building is used to classify types of building use. Simply multiplying the weight of all combustible materials by their energy values and dividing by the floor area under consideration calculates the fire load.

Work with dangerous chemicals is subject to the legislative requirements of the **Dangerous Substances and Explosive Atmospheres Regulations (DSEAR) 2002.** Dangerous substances or preparations include substances that are:

▶ explosive;
▶ oxidizing;
▶ extremely flammable;
▶ highly flammable; or
▶ flammable.

An **explosive atmosphere** is a mixture, under atmospheric conditions, of air and one or more dangerous substances in the form of gases, vapours, mists or dusts in which, after ignition has occurred, combustion spreads to the entire unburned mixture.

Recommended limits for storage of substances within the premises (building):

▶ no more than 50 litres for extremely, highly flammable and those flammable liquids with a flashpoint below the maximum ambient temperature of the workroom/working area; and
▶ no more the 250 litres for other flammable liquids with a higher flashpoint of up to 60°C

Revision exercise

Outline factors to be considered when liaising with the fire authority. (4)

Exam tip

Develop a list that would be helpful to the fire authority if they came to your premises to tackle a fire.

Outline steps to minimise the environmental impact of fire and fire fighting operations

Key revision points

▶ Sources of pollution in the event of a fire: toxic and corrosive smoke, run-off of contaminated fire-fighting water

▶ Legal obligations related to environmental protection in the event of a fire, the role of the Environment Agency or Scottish Environmental Protection Agency or Northern Ireland Environment Agency in the event of a fire, Water Resources Act 1991

▶ Factors to be considered in pre-planning the minimisation of environmental impact of fire

▶ Site and damaged area clean up consideration.

Sources of pollution in the event of a fire: Toxic and corrosive smoke, run-off of contaminated fire-fighting water

Sources of pollution include:

▶ Smoke: may contain harmful products:
  ▷ toxic chemicals;
  ▷ particulates;
  ▷ asbestos; and
  ▷ carbon monoxide.
▶ Run-off of contaminated fire-fighting water. Water or foam used to fight fires at premises where chemicals are used or stored can become contaminated with the chemicals and become hazardous in itself.

Pathways by which pollutants from the site of a fire can enter the water ecosystem:

▶ the surface water drainage system on site;
▶ through the foul drainage system contaminating the sewage works beds; or

170

▶ by water run-off to ground and into brooks, streams and rivers and by airborne contaminants deposited in precipitation.

Legal obligations related to environmental protection in the event of a fire, the role of the Environment Agency or Scottish Environmental Protection Agency or Northern Ireland Environment Agency in the event of a fire, Water Resources Act 1991

National enforcing agencies:

▶ Environment Agency
▶ Scottish Environmental Protection Agency
▶ Northern Ireland Environment Agency

The **Water Resources Act 1991** applies to England and Wales. It applies to surface, ground and coastal waters (up to three miles). Its purpose is to consolidate previous water legislation concerning water resources. It defines the responsibilities of the Environment Agency (previously known as the National Rivers Authority) to prevent the pollution of watercourses and groundwater.

Section 85: Offences of polluting controlled waters

A person contravenes this section if:

▶ He/she causes, or knowingly permits, any poisonous, noxious or polluting matter or any solid waste matter to enter any controlled waters.
▶ He/she causes, or knowingly permits, any matter, other than trade effluent or sewage effluent, to enter controlled waters by being discharged from a drain or sewer in contravention of a prohibition imposed under Section 86 below.

Criminal Liability

▶ S85(1) Water Resources Act 1991 established the general offence of causing, or knowingly permitting, any poisonous, noxious, or polluting matter or any waste to enter controlled waters.

171

Factors to be considered in pre-planning the minimisation of environmental impact of fire

Pollutants may escape from the site into the water environment by a number of pathways. These include:

▶ Direct run-off into nearby watercourses or onto ground, with potential risk to ground waters.
▶ The site's surface water drainage system, either directly or via off-site surface water sewers.
▶ Through atmospheric deposition, such as vapour plumes.
▶ Via the foul drainage system, with pollutants either passing unaltered through a sewage treatment works or affecting the performance of the works, resulting in further environmental damage.

Control measures that could be used to contain fire-fighting water run-off

These include:

▶ Use of bunds;
▶ Use of drain covers, mats and sand bags;
▶ Interceptors;
▶ Sacrificial area and/or trenches;
▶ Diverting and directing the flow of water taking full advantage of the lie of the land; or
▶ Use of a secondary containment reservoir or lagoon and by the use of portable containers or tanks.

Site and damaged area clean up consideration[10]

Procedure should include the following, if appropriate:

▶ Provision of firewater lagoons.
▶ Spills involving hazardous materials should first be contained to prevent spread of the material to other areas.
▶ Availability of emergency equipment – for example, sand bags, dry sand absorbent pads.

- Wherever possible the material should be rendered safe by treating with appropriate chemicals.
- Hazardous materials in a fine dusty form should not be cleared up by dry brushing. Vacuum cleaners should be used in preference, and for toxic materials.
- Treated material should be absorbed onto inert carrier material to allow the material to be cleared up and removed to a safe place for disposal or further treatment as appropriate.
- Waste should not be allowed to accumulate.
- A regular and frequent waste removal procedure should be adopted.

Revision exercise

With regards to the environment, **identify THREE** national enforcing agencies. (3)

Exam tip

Identify the substances that may cause pollution, within your workplace in the event of a fire.

References

1 Building Regulations (2010) *Explanatory Note*. p.53. Available at: http://www.legislation.gov.uk/uksi/2010/2214/pdfs/uksi_20102214_en.pdf
2 Building Regulations (2010) Available at: http://www.legislation.gov.uk/uksi/2010/2214/pdfs/uksi_20102214_en.pdf
3 Available at: http://www.mace.manchester.ac.uk/project/research/structures/strucfire/DataBase/References/ASPE%20publications/ASPE05_An%20industry%20guide%20to%20design%20for%20installation%20of%20fire%20&%20smoke%20resisting%20dampers%20(Grey%20Book).pdf
4 NFPA 92A, Recommended practice for smoke control system, National Fire Protection Association, Quincy, MA, USA (2001).
5 Available at: http://www.canonfire.co.uk/products/fire-detection-alarms/detection-devices/

6 DCLG guide . . .
7 Available at: https://www.ddfire.gov.uk/number-fire-extinguishers-required
8 Approved Document B (2006, revised in 2007, 2010 and 2013)
9 BS 9999 Section 6.
10 Available at: http://www.hse.gov.uk/comah/sragtech/techmeasspill.htm

Safety of people in the event of fire

Learning outcomes

Explain the purpose and requirements of a fire emergency plan ☐

Describe the development and maintenance of a fire evacuation procedure ☐

Outline the perception and behaviour of people in the event of a fire ☐

Outline appropriate training requirements ☐

Explain the purpose and requirements of a fire emergency plan

Key revision points

▶ Purpose of a Fire Emergency Plan
▶ Content of a Fire Emergency Plan
▶ Multi-occupied premises (need to consult/comply with all occupiers)
▶ Compatibility of the emergency plan with the everyday use of the premises

Purpose of a fire emergency plan

The purpose is to ensure all employees, visitors, etc. are aware of the actions to be taken in the event of fire and are safely evacuated from the premises to the assembly point prior to the fire brigade arriving.

Content of a fire emergency plan

The content a fire emergency plan may include:

▶ action people should take in the event of a fire;
▶ action people should take on discovering a fire;
▶ appropriate isolating of machinery and processes;
▶ arrangements for calling the fire and rescue service;
▶ details of assembly points;
▶ details of evacuation procedure;
▶ duties and identities of persons with specific responsibilities;
▶ fire fighting arrangements;
▶ how people will be warned/fire alarm activation procedure;
▶ how the fire service are called and by whom;
▶ liaison with fire service on arrival;
▶ procedures for meeting the fire and rescue service on arrival; and
▶ procedures to help vulnerable people and those with disabilities.

176

Multi-occupied premises (need to consult/comply with all occupiers)

If there is more than one responsible person in any type of premises (e.g. a multi-occupied complex), all must take reasonable steps to co-operate and co-ordinate with each other. All those with some control must co-operate with each other and will need to consider the risk generated by others in the building.

Evacuation procedure for a shared occupancy office building

In multi-occupied premises escape routes should normally be independent of other occupiers – i.e. people should not have to go through another occupier's premises as the route may be secured or obstructed. Where this is not possible, then robust legal agreements should be in place to ensure their availability at all times.

Compatibility of the emergency plan with the everyday use of the premises

The emergency plan will need to be more detailed and compiled only after consultation with other occupiers and other responsible people (e.g. owners) who have control over the building. In most cases a single emergency plan covering the whole building will be necessary.

Revision exercise

Identify the typical content a fire emergency plan. (8)

Exam tip

Read your company's fire emergency plan.

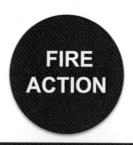

FIRE ACTION

IF YOU DISCOVER A FIRE:
a) Immediately operate the nearest fire alarm call point
b) Attack the fire if possible with the appliances provided but do not take personal risks

IF YOU HEAR THE FIRE ALARM:

c) [   ]

will call the fire brigade immediately by telephone
(Always call the fire brigade immediately to every fire or suspicion of fire)

1. Dial '999'
2. Give the operator your telephone number and ask for FIRE
3. When the fire brigade replies give the call distinctly: Fire at

[   ]

DO NOT replace the receiver until the address has been repeated by the FIRE BRIGADE

d) Leave the building and report to the person in charge of the assembly point

[   ]

USE THE NEAREST AVAILABLE EXIT

Do not stop to collect personal belongings

Never re-enter the building until authorised to do so

Figure 4 Example of a fire action notice, giving brief details of the fire emergency plan

Describe the development and maintenance of a fire evacuation procedure

Key revision points

▶ The purposes of, and essential requirements for, evacuation procedures and drills, alarm evacuation and roll call
▶ Procedures to evacuate vulnerable people and people with disabilities and/or mobility problems
▶ Types of evacuation procedures (staged, phased, horizontal, etc.) and interaction with staged alarm systems
▶ Actions required when evacuating members of the public.

The purposes of, and essential requirements for, evacuation procedures and drills, alarm evacuation and roll call

Once the emergency plan has been developed and training given, it will need to be evaluated to check its effectiveness, by undertaking a fire drill. This should be carried out at least annually.

A well-planned and executed fire drill will confirm understanding of the training and provide helpful information for future training.

The possible objectives of the drill are to:

▶ identify any weaknesses in the evacuation strategy;
▶ test the procedure following any recent alteration or changes to working practices;
▶ familiarise new members of staff with procedures; and
▶ test the arrangements for disabled people.

For both drills and for real fires, a roll call should be carried out as soon as possible at the designated assembly point(s), and/or the fire brigade will receive reports from wardens designated to 'sweep' the premises. In a real evacuation this information will need to be passed to the fire and rescue service on arrival.

The maintenance of a fire evacuation procedure may include:

▶ Checks of fire resisting doors, walls and partitions – are they damaged?
▶ Checks of escape routes – are they kept clear?
▶ Checks of exit doors – are they damaged?
▶ Checks of fire safety signs – can they be seen?
▶ Maintenance regime for the fire warning system:
  ▷ Weekly
  ▷ Annually
▶ Maintenance regime for the emergency lighting system:
  ▷ Weekly
  ▷ Monthly
  ▷ Annually
▶ Maintenance of the fire fighting equipment:
  ▷ Weekly
  ▷ Annually.

Procedures to evacuate vulnerable people and people with disabilities and/or mobility problems

Need to consider those who have and/or are:

▶ sleeping occupants;
▶ disabled occupants:
  ▷ mobility impaired,
  ▷ mentally impaired,
  ▷ visually impaired,
  ▷ hearing impaired;
▶ occupants in remote areas;
▶ lone workers;
▶ pregnant;
▶ young persons (under 18);
▶ elderly, who need assistance;
▶ those not familiar with the premises; and
▶ non-English speaking.

Types of evacuation procedures (staged, phased, horizontal, etc.) and interaction with staged alarm systems

Types of alarm actions

► Single staged – total
► Two staged – staff interaction with alarm system
► Staff controlled – required when evacuating members of the public.

Types of evacuation

► Progressive horizontal – residential care/hospitals
► Progressive vertical – multi-story buildings; for example:

1 The floor of origin of the fire and the floor immediately above
2 The next two floors above
3 The remaining floors in groups of two working up the building
4 Floors in groups of two below the floor of origin working downwards.

Regular fire drills should be carried out to both support the training given and test that procedures work appropriately.

Actions required when evacuating members of the public

The responsible person will need to ensure that all fire safety provisions are in place and that fire wardens etc. have received additional training when members of the public are within the premises. Constant checks may be needed while the public are present, and again after they have left.

Revision exercise

Identify different types of vulnerable persons that need to be considered when developing an emergency evacuation plan. (8)

Exam tip

Consider the vulnerable persons that are in your place of work – are there sufficient arrangements in place?

Outline the perception and behaviour of people in the event of a fire

Key revision points

▶ Principles of sensory perception
▶ Effect of time pressure and stress on the decision making process during fire emergencies
▶ Likely behaviour of individuals responsible for others during a fire
▶ Effect of different behaviours on fire and evacuation
▶ Crowd movement (individuals and in groups): how crowd flow can cause danger and prohibit safe escape, modification of crowd flow by physical design and messages
▶ Measures to overcome behavioural problems.

Principles of sensory perception

The way in which people perceive risk is a mixture of an individual's:

▶ skills;
▶ knowledge;
▶ attitudes;
▶ training;
▶ experience;
▶ personality;
▶ memory; and
▶ ability to process sensory information.

Evacuation has four distinct phases:

Phase 1 Alert time from fire initiation to detection/recognition – via the fire alarm, smell of smoke or feel the heat.

Phase 2 Pre-movement time taken by behaviour that diverts an individual from the escape route/s – the individuals may not recognise the fire threat, i.e. think it is 'another' false alarm. They may not perceive the risk due to drugs/alcohol, or they may have a tendency to panic, etc. Response may be different due to the type of alarm; a verbal alarm is considered more effective than beeping alarm.

Phase 3 Travel time to physically get to an exit – this may be affected by a person's physical and mental abilities.

Phase 4 Flow time – i.e. how long it takes for the occupants to move through the various stages of the escape route.

Effect of time pressure and stress on the decision-making process during fire emergencies

Potential hindrances that could have an impact on action taken in the event of a fire include:

▶ Difficulties of spatial orientation and way finding in large and complex locations may affect individuals with dyslexia or other leaning needs.
▶ Patterns of exit choice in fire emergencies may cause problems – for example, if there is poor signage within the premises.
▶ Implications of exit choice behaviour in designing for fire safety – i.e. it is common practice to exit the building via the route that someone entered. Employees and visitors should be made aware of alternate fire exit routes.
▶ People do not generally respond to a single stimulus and often wait for others to respond.

Likely behaviour of individuals responsible for others during a fire

Those who are responsible for children or patients – for example,

▶ parents,
▶ elder siblings,
▶ nurses, and
▶ teachers –

will likely respond to an emergency situation (a fire) by going to help the children in their care without regard for their own safety or the evacuation procedures that are in place.

Effect of different human behaviours on fire and evacuation

Factors that make people slow to respond in a fire:

▶ A desire to finish a task.
▶ A lack of understanding of the hazards resulting from smoke or how the fire might spread.
▶ A poor perception of the danger involved.
▶ Fright and panic can cause people to freeze.
▶ From curiosity – i.e. would seek to gain a view of the fire.
▶ Locating family members or friends.
▶ Tendency to ignore alarms – believing it to be a false alarm.
▶ Wanting to collect belongings.
▶ Language problems and lack of training may also be issues.

Crowd movement (individuals and in groups): How crowd flow can cause danger and prohibit safe escape, modification of crowd flow by physical design and messages

The problems associated with the behaviour of individuals in the event of fire are increased when large numbers of people are gathered together – i.e. in crowds. The behaviour of individuals in a

184

crowd often differs from when those same people are by themselves or in smaller groups. For example:

▶ Individuals in a crowd can be greatly influenced by the actions of others.
▶ Individuals in a crowd are more likely to be prone to panic.
▶ Individuals' emotions may be heightened in a crowd.

Modification of crowd flow can be addressed by physical design of escape routes and procedural measures.

Physical design of escape routes to be considered for crowds include:

▶ clear signage;
▶ wider emergency routes;
▶ one way systems; and
▶ alternate routes.

Procedural measures to be considered for crowds include:

▶ Additional fire wardens to aid people to a place of safety.
▶ Automated voice instructions rather than beeping/siren fire alarms.

Measures to overcome behavioural problems

Factors to consider when trying to overcome behavioural problems include:

▶ Ensuring escape routes are kept clear.
▶ Having well-practiced drills.
▶ Implementing measures to assist vulnerable people and people with disabilities and/or mobility problems.
▶ Including contingency to deal with sleeping people within the evacuation strategy.
▶ Setting clear roles and responsibilities.
▶ Using clear alarms.

The use of coded messages for stewards will reduce problems of panic and a planned emergency strategy.

Revision exercise

Describe the FOUR distinct phases of an evacuation. (8)

Exam tip

Do you know the alternate fire exit routes from your place of work, or other places you visit?

Outline appropriate training requirements

Key revision points

▶ Fire safety training information for employees/workers, temporary, agency staff and volunteers etc.
▶ Need for competent people to assist employers
▶ Individual roles and responsibilities in an emergency
▶ Employees/workers with management/supervisory roles

Fire safety training information for employees/workers, temporary, agency staff and volunteers, etc.

All employees/workers, temporary, agency staff and volunteers, etc. should know:

▶ how to summon the fire brigade;
▶ how to warn others – operation of the fire-warning apparatus;
▶ the location and use of escape routes;
▶ the procedure for assisting visitors or members of the public from the workplace;
▶ the location of the fire assembly point; and
▶ how to use the fire equipment provided.

186

Fire Marshal/Warden should know:

▶ theory of fire (triangle);

▶ fire risk assessment;

▶ positioning for alarms, call points, lighting, extinguishers, etc.;

▶ inspection of equipment: alarms, call points, lighting, extinguishers, etc.;

▶ evacuation training; and

▶ practical use of fire fighting equipment.

Those requiring specific training will include:

▶ Fire wardens/marshals;

▶ Fire risk assessors;

▶ Fire extinguisher technicians;

▶ Sprinkler system technicians;

▶ Fire alarm technicians;

▶ Emergency lighting technicians; and

▶ Those who will use evacuation chairs/slides.

Training will need to include specific knowledge of fire and emergency procedures for their places of work.

Need for competent people to assist employers

NEBOSH qualification matches competency criteria for fire risk assessors

The NEBOSH National Certificate in Fire Safety and Risk Management 2013 syllabus and means of assessment has taken into account current developments in health and safety, fire safety, risk management and vocational assessment. The syllabus has been mapped to the 'Competency Criteria for Fire Risk Assessors' that has been produced by the Fire Risk Assessment Competency Council.

Professional bodies that operate schemes for fire risk assessors

▶ Institute of Fire Prevention Officers (IFPO)

▶ Institute of Fire Safety Managers (IFSM)

▶ Institution of Fire Engineers (IFE)
▶ Warrington Certification Ltd.

Individual roles and responsibilities in an emergency

Those appointed as fire wardens/marshals will have specific duties:

▶ **In the event of a fire, their role is:**
  ▷ Ensuring everyone in the building is accounted for.
  ▷ Ensuring the Fire Brigade has been called.
  ▷ Liaising with the Fire Brigade on their arrival.
  ▷ Coordinating contingency planning if the situation requires it.
  ▷ Ensuring the building is safe before anyone is allowed to re-enter.

▶ **When there is no fire, their role may include checking:**
  ▷ fire resisting doors, walls and partitions;
  ▷ escape routes;
  ▷ exit doors;
  ▷ fire safety signs;
  ▷ fire warning system (weekly checks);
  ▷ fire emergency lighting system (weekly and/or monthly checks);
  ▷ fire doors (weekly and/or monthly checks); and
  ▷ fire fighting equipment (weekly check).

Employees/workers with management/ supervisory roles

Fire wardens have roles for both emergency situations and for normal day-to-day activities.

For emergency situations for fire wardens:

▶ Sweep through their allocated area, turning off equipment and closing doors/windows in passing but not delaying their own escape unduly, while encouraging people to leave via the nearest fire escape route. The fire warden should normally be the last person off the floor.
▶ Checking all accessible rooms including toilets and offices to make sure people are beginning their evacuation.

188

▶ Checking any refuge in their area in case someone is waiting for assistance to evacuate.

▶ Reporting to the person in charge of the evacuation, at the assembly area or just outside the building, to advise that the area is clear (or to report anyone who can't or won't leave the building).

▶ To assist the officer in charge with crowd control, verbally encouraging people towards the assembly area.

▶ To take part in any post-alarm de-briefing to identify any shortcomings in the evacuation procedures.

▶ Only if it is safe to do so AND practical training has been given – to tackle small fires.

Normal activities for fire wardens:

Day-to-day role includes checking that (within the area they are allocated):

▶ No issues arise with regard to general fire safety of the area, building or floor the warden has been allocated.

▶ There are no combustible materials and/or obstructions in corridors or walkways.

▶ Escape routes are kept free of obstructions.

▶ Fire doors are not tied, propped or wedged open where they should not be.

▶ Final exit doors are not obstructed.

▶ Fire extinguishers are where they should be and no obvious misuse or defect has occurred.

▶ Fire call points and emergency lighting units are not damaged.

▶ Fire alarm panel is in normal operation.

Weekly/monthly role includes:

▶ Testing the fire alarm via a different call point each week.

▶ Testing the emergency lighting (this may be done in part weekly, to ensure all lighting is checked once per month).

General duties of employees at work:[1]

▶ take reasonable care for the safety of themselves and of other relevant persons who may be affected by their acts or omissions at work;

189

▶ co-operate with their employer, with regard to fire safety measures;

▶ inform their employer of any serious and immediate danger to safety; and

▶ inform their employer of any shortcoming in the employer's protection arrangements for fire safety.

Fire safety information should include:

▶ What to do in the event of a fire
▶ Location of:
  ▷ Assembly point(s)
  ▷ Fire extinguishers
  ▷ Call points
  ▷ Emergency exits
▶ Knowledge of the 'sound' of the fire alarm
▶ Knowledge of special evacuation arrangements for people with disabilities.

Revision exercise

Outline the general duties of employees, with regards to fire safety. (8)

Exam tip

Consider the roles you have at work with regards to fire safety.

Reference

1 The Regulatory Reform (Fire Safety) Order 2005.

Fire risk assessment

Explain the aims and objectives of fire risk assessments

Key revision points

▶ Meaning of hazard and risk in relation to a fire
▶ Criteria for a 'suitable and sufficient risk assessment'
▶ Objectives of fire risk assessments
▶ Distinction between different types of fire incident.

Meaning of hazard and risk in relation to a fire

Following definitions are taken from PAS79:2012:

▶ **Fire hazard:** source, situation or unsafe act with potential to result in a fire.

> Examples of fire hazards include ignition sources, accumulation of waste that could be subject to ignition and disposal of a lit cigarette close to combustible materials.

▶ **Fire risk:** combination of the likelihood of the occurrence of fire and consequence(s) (number and severity of injuries) likely to be caused by a fire.

> Examples of relevant consequences of a fire are those involving injury to people as opposed to damage to property.

Criteria for a 'suitable and sufficient fire risk assessment'

A fire risk assessment should:

▶ Identify the significant risks and ignore the trivial ones.
▶ Identify and prioritize the measures required to comply with any relevant statutory provisions.
▶ Remain appropriate to the nature of the work and valid over a reasonable period of time.

▶ Identify the risk arising from, or in connection with, the work.
▶ The level of detail should be proportionate to the risk.

Examples of when a fire risk assessment is not a 'suitable and sufficient risk assessment':

In 2013 the fire service welcomed a guilty verdict for a Goldthorpe supermarket owner who repeatedly ignored warnings to comply with safety laws. The owner was found guilty at Sheffield Magistrates Court of failing to comply with five articles of the Regulatory Reform (Fire Safety) Order 2005. A £1,300 fine was handed down by magistrates for failing to comply with an enforcement notice and failing to have a suitable and sufficient risk assessment. He was also ordered to pay £1,800 costs.[1]

An external fire risk assessor and a hotel manager were both jailed for eight months for multiple breaches of the Regulatory Reform (Fire Safety) Order 2005. During the trial, the Judge said that the time had come to send out a message to those who conduct fire risk assessments and to hoteliers who are prepared to put profit before safety. The offences related to failing to provide suitable risk assessments, and failures of the responsible person, including inadequate fire doors at the premises that compromised exit routes.[2]

Objectives of fire risk assessments

The primary objective of a fire risk assessment is the protection of life and harm to individuals (**moral duty**).

Additional objectives include **legal** compliance and **financial** factors (for the business and/or organisation) in addition to **environmental** factors.

Human harm

- death;
- personal injury; or
- psychological harm.

Legal effects

- prosecution: fines and imprisonment.

Financial/economic effects

- damage to premises;
- damage to products and stock;
- loss of business reputation; or
- local transport disruption.

Environmental effects

- flora and fauna damage; or
- pollution of waterways.

Safety measures and management policies necessary to reduce the risk to persons from fire will need to be introduced. This may be in the form of an action list, on completion of the fire risk assessment, and it will also include the current fire safety policy and procedures.

Distinction between different types of fire incident

Work injury

Is any accident resulting in physical injury to a person whilst at work (or at a place of study where students are concerned) – for example, someone injured falling over during a fire drill?

Work ill health

Is any condition believed to be attributable to work or the workplace – for example, illness caused by inhalation of toxic smoke during a fire.

Near miss

Is an undesired event or condition where no injury, ill health, damages or other loss occurs – for example, failure of fire alarm system.

Dangerous occurrence

These are serious incidents (see RIDDOR Schedule 2) – for example, a fire or explosion or ignition at a site where the manufacture or storage of explosives requires a license or registration.

Fire incident

Are incidents where an actual fire occurs.

Revision exercise

(a) **State** the meaning of:
   (i) Fire hazard (1)
   (ii) Fire risk (2)
(b) **Outline** the meaning of the term 'suitable and sufficient fire risk assessment'. (5)

Exam tip

When answering a question that requires you to write the meaning, develop your answer as short sentences. The number you need to include will be indicated in the form of the possible marks. Remember each sentence needs to refer to something different to gain all the marks.

Outline the principles and practice of fire risk assessments including principles of prevention

---

Key revision points

▶ Identification of laws, regulations and guidance to be considered
▶ Identifying fire hazards
▶ Methods of identifying hazards
▶ Identify people at risk
▶ Evaluation of risk and the adequacy of existing fire safety measures
▶ Evaluate the likelihood that a fire may occur
▶ Evaluate the hazards to people in the event of a fire
▶ Evaluate the consequence to people from a fire starting
▶ Risk reduction
▶ Avoid or reduce hazards that may cause a fire
▶ Put in place fire safety measures to reduce the risk to persons from fire
▶ Principles of prevention
▶ Recording significant findings: format, information to be recorded
▶ Reviewing the fire risk assessment, reasons for review
▶ Sources of information that could be consulted.

Identification of laws, regulations and guidance to be considered

The legal requirement in the UK for undertaking a fire risk assessment:

England and Wales

▶ Regulatory Reform Fire Safety Order 2005
▶ The person responsible for fire safety is called the **'Responsible Person'.**

Scotland

▶ Fire Safety (Scotland) Regulations 2006
▶ The person responsible for fire safety is called the **'Duty Holder'.**

Northern Ireland

▶ Fire and Rescue Services (Northern Ireland) Order 2006
▶ The person responsible for fire safety is called the **'Appropriate Person'.**

Guidance to be considered includes the Department for Communities and Local Government (DCLG 2005) Fire Guides.[3] (See Element 1 for details.)

For example, the meaning of Responsible Person is defined in Article 3 of the Regulatory Reform Fire Safety Order 2005 as:

(a) in relation to a workplace, the employer, if the workplace is to any extent under his control;

(b) in relation to any premises not falling within paragraph (a)—

(I) the person who has control of the premises (as occupier or otherwise) in connection with the carrying on by him of a trade, business or other undertaking (for profit or not); or

(II) the owner, where the person in control of the premises does not have control in connection with the carrying on by that person of a trade, business or other undertaking.

The Responsible Person can be either an individual or an entity such as a limited company.

Identifying fire hazards (fire prevention)

Fire prevention (aka *process fire safety*)

This focuses on the three elements of the fire triangle (**oxygen, ignition and fuel**), with the aim of preventing them uniting – to avoid a fire occurring in the first place! This includes maintenance programmes in place for fire hazards – for example, electrical mains, portable appliances, heating, cooking, the storage of flammable liquids, flammable gases, combustible and/or explosive materials.

The fire triangle principle illustrates that to start a fire the three components need to be present, and a chemical reaction needs to take place: ignition source, fuel and oxygen. These three factors should be considered when identifying the fire hazards.

The following are examples of possible ignition sources within the work place:[4]

▶ electrical sources of ignition;
▶ smoking;
▶ arson;
▶ portable heaters and heating installations;
▶ cooking;
▶ lightning;
▶ housekeeping;
▶ hazards introduced by outside contractors and building works;
▶ dangerous substances; and
▶ process fire hazards:
    ▷ hot work (welding, grinding, etc.),
    ▷ overheating of machinery, and
    ▷ spontaneous ignition of oil and solvent soaked materials.

The following are examples of possible fuel sources within the work place:

▶ paper and cardboard;
▶ furniture, fixtures and fittings;
▶ structural materials;
▶ wall and ceiling linings;
▶ flammable liquids;
▶ flammable gases (cylinders and piped gas);
▶ flammable vapours;
▶ combustible materials; and
▶ explosive materials.

The following are examples of possible oxygen sources within the work place:

▶ heating and ventilation systems (HAVS);
▶ natural ventilation (open windows);
▶ oxidizing materials;

▶ oxygen condensers; and

▶ oxygen cylinders.

When undertaking a fire risk assessment, addressing **Fire Prevention,** the following questions should be considered:

Ignition	What potential causes of ignition were not controlled during the fire risk assessment? For example, was it noted that: ▶ There was visible evidence of damage to electrical mains and/or appliances? ▶ Employees were smoking in a non-designated area and/or inside the building? Within this section, further testing and maintenance is to be documented. Is there an external maintenance programme in place for fire hazards – for example, electrical mains, portable appliances, heating, cooking, etc.?
Fuel	▶ Is there an acceptable level of risk from housekeeping? ▶ Is there a risk from flammable liquids, flammable gases, combustible and/or explosive materials?
Oxygen	▶ Is there additional risk, which is not adequately controlled, from heating and ventilation systems (HAVS), oxidizing materials, etc.?

Identifying fire hazards (fire precautions)

Fire precautions (general fire safety)

This focuses on reducing the risk of fire on the premises and the risk of the spread of fire on the premises. It assesses means of escape, fire fighting, fire detection and warning, maintenance programmes and management systems (training, drills, details for and when fire risk assessments should be reviewed, etc.). This includes Emergency Fire Safety Arrangements – i.e. what to do in the event of a fire.

The definition of general fire precautions is included in local legislation – for example, in Article 4 of the Regulatory

Reform Fire Safety Order 2005 – that outlines the general fire precautions:[5]

(a) measures to reduce the risk of fire on the premises and the risk of the spread of fire on the premises;

(b) measures in relation to the means of escape from the premises;

(c) measures for securing that, at all material times, the means of escape can be safely and effectively used;

(d) measures in relation to the means for fighting fires on the premises;

(e) measures in relation to the means for detecting fire on the premises and giving warning in case of fire on the premises; and

(f) measures in relation to the arrangements for action to be taken in the event of fire on the premises, including – (i) measures relating to the instruction and training of employees; and (ii) measures to mitigate the effects of the fire.

When undertaking a fire risk assessment, addressing **Fire Precautions,** the following questions should be considered:

Means of detection	▶ What type of detection system is in place? ▶ Does it meet the relevant national standards for the type of premises and number of people?
Means of escape	▶ Do travel distances meet relevant national standards? ▶ Are there breaches within compartments and/or voids included? ▶ Is there sufficient emergency escape lighting? ▶ Is there sufficient fire signage? ▶ Is there suitable fire fighting equipment? ▶ Are fire doors adequate?
Maintenance programmes	▶ Is there internal testing of the fire safety measures (including fire alarm, emergency lighting, fire fighting equipment, doors, etc.)? ▶ Is there an external maintenance programme in place for the fire safety measures (including fire alarm, emergency lighting, fire fighting equipment, etc.)?

Management systems	▶ Is there a suitable fire safety management system in place, including relevant documentation – for example, fire safety policy, log book and records of previous visits from Fire Authority?
	▶ Is there an adequate level of training and sufficient number of fire drills being undertaken?

Methods of identifying hazards

Identifying fire hazards in the workplace can be achieved by undertaking a:

▶ fire risk assessment;
▶ workplace inspection;
▶ general risk assessment; or
▶ job/task analysis; etc.

The primary way will involve looking for specific hazards identified above – for example, are there any electric hazards (damaged equipment, sockets, misuse of appliances, etc.) that could start a fire?

Identify people at risk

All relevant persons should be considered when undertaking a fire risk assessment.

Relevant persons are

▶ any person who is, or may be, lawfully on the premises; or
▶ any person in the immediate vicinity of the premises who is at risk from a fire on the premises.

This will include employees, contractors, visitors, cleaners, volunteers, etc.

Vulnerable persons are those especially at risk from fire, including:

▶ sleeping occupants;
▶ disabled occupants:
  ▷ mobility impaired,

▷ mentally impaired,

▷ visually impaired,

▷ hearing impaired;

▶ occupants in remote areas;

▶ lone workers;

▶ pregnant women;

▶ young persons (under 18);

▶ elderly, who need assistance;

▶ those not familiar with the premises; and

▶ non-English speaking.

Evaluation of risk and the adequacy of existing fire safety measures

For any significant **Fire Prevention** hazards, identified suitable control measures need to be introduced.

Evaluate the likelihood that a fire may occur

The likelihood that a fire may occur can be evaluated using the following:

Table 3 Likelihood of fire (based on PAS 79:2012)

High	Lack of adequate controls applied to one or more significant fire hazards, such as to result in significant increase in likelihood of fire
Medium	Normal fire hazards (e.g. potential ignition sources) for this type of occupancy, within fire hazards generally subject to appropriate controls (other than minor shortcomings)
Low	Unusually low likelihood of fire as a result of negligible potential sources of ignition

Evaluate the consequence to people from a fire starting

The fire risk assessor will need to identify the likelihood of a fire and the potential consequences of that fire. This could be accomplished using the following three tables:

Table 4 Consequence of a fire (based on PAS 79:2012)

High	Significant potential for serious injury or death of one or more occupants
Medium	Outbreak of fire could foreseeably result in injury (including serious injury) of one or more occupants, but it is unlikely to involve multiple fatalities
Low	Outbreak of fire unlikely to result in serious injury or death of any occupant (other than an occupant sleeping in a room in which a fire occurs)

Using the above likelihood of fire and consequence of fire it is possible to evaluate the level of risk.

Table 5 Fire risk level estimator (adapted from PAS 79:2012)

Likelihood of fire	Potential consequences of fire		
	Low	**Medium**	**High**
Low	Low	Medium	Medium
Medium	Medium	Medium	High
High	Medium	High	High

An alternate method can be used – the more traditional health and safety quantitative approach.

Table 6 5 × 5 matrix

Consequence					
5	5	10	15	20	25
4	4	8	12	16	20
3	3	6	9	12	15
2	2	4	6	8	10
1	1	2	3	4	5
			Likelihood		

Likelihood × Severity

1. Very unlikely / improbable	1. Insignificant – no first aid needed
2. Unlikely / remote	2. Minor – first aid
3. Fairly likely / possible	3. Moderate – hospital
4. Likely / probable	4. Major – hospital
5. Very likely	5. Catastrophic – death / disabling

Risk reduction

There are various methods used for risk reduction – for example, the general hierarchy of control:

- ▶ **eliminate** the hazard;
- ▶ **substitute** with less hazardous materials, processes, operations or equipment;
- ▶ use **engineering** controls;
- ▶ use **administrative** controls (including safety signs, etc.); and
- ▶ provide and ensure use of adequate **personal protective equipment**.

When considering risk reduction for fire safety, the priority is the prevention of the fire occurring – i.e. keeping ignition and fuel sources apart and, where practical, preventing additional oxygen sources interfering with any potential combustion process.

The following priority matrix can be used to help justify action plans for risk reduction.

---

1 Breach of legislation and/or guidance and risk of death or serious injury

2 Breach of legislation and/or guidance but no risk of death or serious injury

3 No breach – good practice

    A Immediately – within one month

    B Short term – within three months

    C Medium term – within six months

    D Long term – within one year and/or time of refurbishment or upgrading

---

Put in place fire safety measures to reduce the risk to persons from fire

The following are examples of typical fire safety issues that may be present in a workplace.

204

Factors that increase the risk of fire and smoke spreading:

1 holes in walls;
2 vents not closing in the event of a fire;
3 doors that don't close;
4 ceiling has voids;
5 walls are constructed of materials that will promote the spread of fire; or
6 air conditioning duct work allowing spread of smoke.

Factors that increase the risk of persons from fire:

1 poor housekeeping that blocks fire exits;
2 poor housekeeping that creates a build-up of combustible material;
3 locked fire exits;
4 alarm unable to be heard in busy workplace;
5 alarm unable to be heard due to faulty siren;
6 call point inaccessible;
7 lack of awareness of what to do in the event of a fire;
8 fire doors propped open by wooden chock;
9 emergency lighting not working;
10 insufficient emergency lighting working;
11 fire safety signs unable to be seen;
12 insufficient number of fire extinguishers;
13 no maintenance of fire safety equipment – therefore may be faulty;
14 no co-ordination with other companies in the premises;
15 means of escape not wide enough for number of people in premises; or
16 not enough exits for number of people in premises.

Practical exercise – complete the following

For each issue, a suitable practical or procedural control measure should be introduced:

Controls for fire and smoke spreading

1
2

3
4
5
6

Controls for persons being harmed by fire

1
2
3
4
5
6
7
8
9
10
11
12
13
14
15
16

Principles of prevention

The **principles of prevention** are identified in the Regulatory Reform Fire Safety Order 2005, Schedule 1, part 3, as:

(a) Avoiding risk;

(b) Evaluating the risks which cannot be avoided;

(c) Combating the risks at source;

(d) Adapting to technical progress;

(e) Replacing the dangerous by the non-dangerous or less dangerous;

(f) Developing a coherent overall prevention policy which covers technology, organisation of work and the influence of factors relating to the working environment;

(g) Giving collective protective measures priority over individual protective measures; and

(h) Giving appropriate instructions to employees.

Recording significant findings: Format, information to be recorded

The format for a fire risk assessment may vary from one organisation to another.

The following is the five-step approach from the DCLG guides:

Step 1 Identify Fire Hazards

Step 2 Identify People at Risk

Step 3 Evaluate, Remove, Reduce and Protect from Risk

Step 4 Record, Plan, Instruct, Inform and Train

Step 5 Keep assessment under review and revise where necessary.

Other methodologies use different systems – for example, PAS79:2012, developed by Collin Todd, has nine steps (BSI, 2012:26):

Step 1 Obtain relevant information about the premises

Step 2 Identification of fire hazards

Step 3 Assessment of likelihood of a fire

Step 4 Determine the physical protection measures

Step 5 Determine relevant information – fire safety management

Step 6 Make a (subjective) assessment of the likely consequences to occupants in the event of fire

Step 7 Make an assessment of the fire risk and decide if the fire risk is tolerable

Step 8 Formulate an action plan

Step 9 Review of the fire risk assessment is necessary after a period of time.

Reviewing the fire risk assessment, reasons for review

The reasons for reviewing a fire risk assessment are similar to when the fire safety policy (and health and safety risk assessment and policy) would need to be reviewed – for example, if there is:

▶ a change in the number of relevant persons;
▶ a lapse of time (e.g. one year);
▶ a result of identified shortcomings in previous risk assessment/ policy;
▶ any alterations to the building;
▶ any changes to work procedures (e.g. introducing hot work)
▶ change of storage or use of flammable liquids / flammable gases (cylinders and piped gas) / combustible materials / explosive materials;
▶ introduction of new equipment that increases the level of risk;
▶ new legislative, or guidance, changes;
▶ significant changes to furniture, fixtures and fittings/structural materials/wall and ceiling linings; and
▶ following a fire and/or enforcement action.

Sources of information that could be consulted

External documents that may be referred to during a fire risk assessment may include:

▶ Local legislation (building and fire);
▶ National guidance documents (Department for Communities and Local Government guides, Approved Documents, etc.);
▶ British Standards Institute (BSI) documents;
▶ The Confederation of Fire Protection Associations in Europe documents;
▶ ⌐ᴖean Fire and Security Group documents;
▶ ⌐ᴖ Protection Association documents; and
▶ / of British Insurers documents.

See learning outcome 1.1 – Outline the main sources of external fire safety information and the principles of their application – for an extended list.

Internal documents that may be referred to during a fire risk assessment may include:

▶ accident / incident log / RIDDOR reports;
▶ fire log book;
▶ fire maintenance records;
▶ fire plan;
▶ health and safety file;
▶ old fire certificate documentation (if available);
▶ operator and machine manuals;
▶ Portable Appliance Tests (PAT) records/electrical checks – installations, etc.;
▶ previous incidents;
▶ previous risk assessments;
▶ training records; and
▶ visitor register(s).

Revision exercise

Outline reasons why a fire risk assessment or fire safety policy would need to be reviewed, assuming that there has not been a fire. (8)

Exam tip

Read your companies fire safety documentation.

Outline matters to be considered in a risk assessment of dangerous substances

---

Key revision points

Matters to be considered in a risk assessment of dangerous substances.

Matters to be considered in a risk assessment of dangerous substances

Factors to be considered when undertaking a risk assessment for dangerous substances include:

▶ Information which may be needed to complete the assessment with regard to:
  ▷ Material Safety Data Sheets of the substances
  ▷ Manufacturers information – with regards to storage, use and disposal.
▶ Arrangements for safe handling, storage and disposal.
▶ Details of the quantities to be stored and used.
▶ Hazardous properties of the substance – e.g.:
  ▷ explosive;
  ▷ oxidizing;
  ▷ extremely flammable;
  ▷ highly flammable; or
  ▷ flammable.
▶ Recommended limits for storage of substances within the premises (building), with reference to Dangerous Substances and Explosive Atmospheres Regulations (DSEAR) 2002:
  ▷ no more than 50 litres for extremely, highly flammable and those flammable liquids with a flashpoint below the maximum ambient temperature of the workroom/working area; and

▷ no more than 250 litres for other flammable liquids with a higher flashpoint of up to 60°C

▶ Safe working procedures.

▶ Likelihood that an explosive atmosphere will occur.

▶ Likelihood that ignition sources will be present and become active and the effective scale of the anticipated effects.

Factors to be considered with regard to risk assessment of dangerous substances include:

▶ the hazardous properties of the substance;

▶ information on safety provided by the supplier;

▶ the circumstances of the work
(special / technical / organisational measures, the substance and possible interactions, amount of substance, risk presented by combination of substances);

▶ arrangements for safe handling;

▶ the likelihood that an explosive atmosphere will occur;

▶ the likelihood that ignition sources will be present and become active and effective;

▶ the scale of the anticipated effects;

▶ any places which are, or can be, connected via openings to places in which explosive atmospheres may occur; and

▶ any additional information which may be needed to completed the assessment.

Revision exercise

Outline factors to be considered with regards to risk assessment of dangerous substances. (8)

Exam tip

Review Schedule 1 Part 1 of the Regulatory Reform (Fire Safety) Order 2005, then **outline** the key factors. (8)

Found at the end of this element.

Outline measures to be taken to control risk in respect of dangerous substances

Key revision points

Measures to be taken to control risk in respect of dangerous substances.

Measures to be taken to control risk in respect of dangerous substances

Factors to be considered with regard to control risk in respect to dangerous substances include:

- ▶ reduce quantities to a minimum;
- ▶ avoid/minimise the release of a dangerous substance;
- ▶ control the release of a dangerous substance at source;
- ▶ prevent the formation of an explosive atmosphere (including appropriate ventilation);
- ▶ ensure that any release of a dangerous substance which may give rise to risk is suitably collected, safely contained, removed to a safe place, or otherwise rendered safe, as appropriate;
- ▶ avoid ignition sources and electrostatic discharges;
- ▶ segregate incompatible dangerous substances;
- ▶ reduce number of persons exposed to a minimum;
- ▶ provide and maintain fire suppression equipment;
- ▶ provide and maintain explosion pressure relief arrangements;
- ▶ measures to avoid propagation of fires/explosions;
- ▶ ensure premises are designed, constructed and maintained so as to reduce risk; and
- ▶ any hazardous jobs involving dangerous substances are carried out under an appropriate system of work including permit-to-work.

Revision exercise

Outline factors to be considered with regard to control risk in respect of dangerous substances. (8)

Exam tip

Review Regulation 5 of the Dangerous Substances and Explosive Atmosphere Regulations 2002, then **outline** the key factors. (8)

Schedule 1 Part 1 of the Regulatory Reform (Fire Safety) Order 2005.

The matters to be considered in risk assessment in respect of dangerous substances include:

(a) the hazardous properties of the substance;

(b) information on safety provided by the supplier, including information contained in any relevant safety data sheet;

(c) the circumstances of the work, including –

  (i) the special, technical and organisational measures and the substances used and their possible interactions,

  (ii) the amount of the substance involved,

  (iii) where the work will involve more than one dangerous substance, the risk presented by such substances in combination, and

  (iv) the arrangements for the safe handling, storage and transport of dangerous substances and of waste containing dangerous substances;

(d) activities, such as maintenance, where there is the potential for a high level of risk;

(e) the effect of measures which have been or will be taken pursuant to this Order;

(f) the likelihood that an explosive atmosphere will occur and its persistence;

(g) the likelihood that ignition sources, including electrostatic discharges, will be present and become active and effective;

(h) the scale of the anticipated effects;

(i) any places which are, or can be, connected via openings to places in which explosive atmospheres may occur; and

(j) such additional safety information as the responsible person may need in order to complete the assessment.

> Regulation 5 of the Dangerous Substances and Explosive Atmosphere Regulations 2002:

(1) Where a dangerous substance is or is liable to be present at the workplace, the employer shall make a suitable and sufficient assessment of the risks to the employees which arise from that substance.

(2) The risk assessment shall include consideration of –

(a) the hazardous properties of the substance;

(b) information on safety provided by the supplier, including information contained in any relevant safety data sheet;

(c) the circumstances of the work including –

    (i) the work processes and substances used and their possible interactions,

    (ii) the amount of the substance involved,

    (iii) where the work will involve more than one dangerous substance, the risk presented by such substances in combination, and

    (iv) the arrangements for the safe handling, storage and transport of dangerous substances and of waste containing dangerous substances;

(d) activities, such as maintenance, where there is the potential for a high level of risk;

(e) the effect of measures which have been or will be taken pursuant to these Regulations;

(f) the likelihood that an explosive atmosphere will occur and its persistence;

(g) the likelihood that ignition sources, including electrostatic discharges, will be present and become active and effective;

(h) the scale of the anticipated effects of a fire or an explosion;

(i) any places which are or can be connected via openings to places in which explosive atmospheres may occur; and

(j) such additional safety information as the employer may need in order to complete the risk assessment.

(3) The risk assessment shall be reviewed by the employer regularly so as to keep it up to-date and particularly if –

  (a) there is reason to suspect that the risk assessment is no longer valid; or

  (b) there has been a significant change in the matters to which the risk assessment relates including when the workplace, work processes, or organisation of the work undergoes significant changes, extensions or conversions; and where, as a result of the review, changes to the risk assessment are required, those changes shall be made.

(4) Where the employer employs five or more employees, the employer shall record the significant findings of the risk assessment as soon as is practicable after that assessment is made, including in particular –

  (a) the measures which have been or will be taken by him pursuant to these Regulations;

  (b) sufficient information to show that the workplace and work processes are designed, operated and maintained with due regard for safety and that, in accordance with the Provision and Use of Work Equipment Regulations 1998(a), adequate arrangements have been made for the safe use of work equipment; and

  (c) where an explosive atmosphere may occur at the workplace and subject to the transitional provisions in regulation 17(1) to (3), sufficient information to show –

    (i) those places which have been classified into zones pursuant to regulation 7(1),

    (ii) equipment which is required for, or helps to ensure, the safe operation of equipment located in places classified as hazardous pursuant to regulation 7(1),

    (iii) that any verification of overall explosion safety required by regulation 7(4) has been carried out, and

    (iv) the aim of any co-ordination required by regulation 11 and the measures and procedures for implementing it.

(5) No new work activity involving a dangerous substance shall commence unless –

(a) an assessment has been made, and

(b) the measures required by these Regulations have been implemented.

References

1 Available at: http://www.syfire.gov.uk/2975.asp

2 Available at: http://www.ifsecglobal.com/fire-risk-assessor-and-hotel-manager-jailed-for-fire-safety-offences-updated-11–07–11/

3 Department for Communities and Local Government Fire Guides Available at: https://www.gov.uk/government/collections/fire-safety-law-and-guidance-documents-for-business

4 British Standards Institute (BSI) (2012) *PAS79: 2012 Fire Risk Assessment: Guidance and a Recommended Methodology*. London: BSI. Available at: http://shop.bsigroup.com/ProductDetail/?pid=000000000030251919

5 Great Britain (2005) *Regulatory Reform (Fire Safety) Order 2005*. London: The Stationery Office. Available at: http://www.legislation.gov.uk/uksi/2005/1541/pdfs/uksi_20051541_en.pdf

Specimen answers to NEBOSH examination questions

Introduction

This chapter is only relevant to those readers who are due to sit for NEBOSH examinations.

The accompanying textbook to this Revision Guide – *Fire Safety and Risk Management* – gives detailed advice on studying for NEBOSH examinations and the NEBOSH guide, 'Guide to the NEBOSH National Certificate in Fire Safety and Risk Management', provides advice on the practical assessment. To gain the full benefit from this section of the Revision Guide, those chapters of the textbook should also be read. But full success in the examinations is only likely to be achieved if a good examination technique is adopted.

Features of a good examination technique

A. Mnemonics

The use of mnemonics during your revision period can be very helpful in the examination. A mnemonic can be a sentence or a word that enables a person to remember a list of items – for example, the colours of the rainbow (red, orange, yellow, green, blue, indigo and violet) can be remembered by the sentence 'Richard of York Gained Battles in Vain'. Similarly, the main factors in a manual handling assessment can be remembered by the word TILE – Task, Individual, Load and Environment.

The best mnemonics are those which students have devised for themselves. The reader is advised to invent his or her own set of mnemonics based on familiar words or sentences. Some examples of useful mnemonics are given below.

1. Management of health and safety

Elements in HSG65	Personal factors	Common topics in the management paper
Plan	**s**elf-interest	**s**afety culture
Do	**h**earing / memory loss	**t**raining
Check	**e**xperience	**r**isk assessment
Act	**a**ge	**i**nformation
	training level	**m**aintenance
	health	**s**upervision
		safe system of work

SHEATH and **STRIMSS** are stand-alone words. (STRIMMS was devised by a student from the horticultural industry.) The reader should devise a suitable sentence to link the initial letters PDCA of HSG 65.

2. Controlling workplace hazards

Risk assessment stages (inc. COSHH and noise)	Machine hazards	Machine guarding
assess the hazards	**e**ntanglement	**f**ixed or fixed distance
control the risks	**n**ips	**i**nterlocked
monitor the controls	**t**raps	**a**djustable
inform employees	**i**mpact	**t**rip devices
record and review the assessment	**c**ontact or cutting	
	ejection	

218

ACMIR can be remembered by 'All Colours Must Include Red'. **ENTICE** and **FIAT** are stand-alone words.

It is very important to stress that a mnemonic is only an aid to memory, and not all the elements in a mnemonic may be relevant to a particular question. Where all or parts of a mnemonic are relevant to a question, you will need to expand on it in your answer.

For example, if the mnemonic, such as STRIMSS, reminds you that 'training and information' are relevant to the question, you should add a brief description of the training and information that you have in mind. Very few marks can be awarded for simply stating 'training and information'.

B. Use of personal experience

The NEBOSH course covers much factual material, which many students find difficult to remember. It is easier to remember this material if it can be related to personal experience and one's own workplace. For example, most workplaces have some hazardous substances present, even if only as cleaning materials. These can be used to illustrate an answer involving hazardous substances (provided that the reference is relevant to the question!). Always try to use familiar examples of hazards and controls when answering examination questions involving those hazards and controls.

C. Simple rules when taking the examination

1 Always arrive at least ten minutes before the start of the examination.
2 Quickly read the whole paper before attempting any question.
3 Start each question on a separate sheet in the answer book and use both sides of the paper. The current NEBOSH answer book has the relevant question number printed on each page of the book.
4 Make brief notes at the beginning of the question page in the answer book.
5 Answer the easiest question first – this may not necessarily be the first one.

6 Read the question carefully and highlight the action verbs (e.g. outline, describe, state etc.). These action verbs are printed in **bold letters** in the question on the examination paper. It is common for candidates to answer the question that they would like to answer rather than the actual one on the examination paper.

7 Answer **all** parts of the question.

8 Attempt **all** questions – you can only get zero marks for an unanswered question.

9 Time is very limited during the examination and answers should be brief and to the point. Do not write all that you know about the topic being questioned or pad out your answer. You should spend no more than 25 minutes on the long answer question (covering about a page and a half) and 8 minutes on each short answer question (normally covering half a page). Most examination failures are caused by not allowing sufficient time to answer all the questions.

10 Finally, the answers should be easy for the examiner to read in terms of layout and standard of writing.

Specimen answers based on NEBOSH examination questions

Some specimen answers are given below to questions based on past NGC1 and FC1 examination questions. Detailed advice is given in the two recommended textbooks that accompany this Revision Guide and in the NEBOSH guide, 'Guide to the NEBOSH National Certificate in Fire Safety and Risk Management'.

It is recommended that, to gain full benefit from the specimen answers, the reader should attempt the questions initially without consulting the answers. The answers given are generally longer than would be expected in the examination because they have covered all possible options that are available in answering a particular question.

Finally, two long answer questions are provided for the NGC1 course because candidates often have more difficulty with this paper.

Practical example: NEBOSH-style question

The following question shows a practical example of each of the command words that are used by NEBOSH (answering a non-health and safety question).

Question

(a) **Identify** types of fruit. (2)

(b) **Give** an example of a fruit that would not be used in a fruit salad. (1)

(c) **Outline** steps to make a fruit salad. (2)

(d) **Describe** a banana. (2)

(e) **Explain** the benefits of eating five fruit and/or vegetables per day. (1)

The following shows a model answers to the above EIGHT-mark question:

(a)
- ▶ Apple;
- ▶ Pear;
- ▶ Kiwi;
- ▶ Orange.

(b)
- ▶ Tomato.

(c)
- ▶ Wash fruit that does not need to be peeled.
- ▶ Cut the fruit into small pieces.
- ▶ Place the pieces into a large bowl.

(d)
- ▶ The bottom end is narrowed; the top has a thick stem, attaching the fruit to the stalk.
- ▶ Ranges from about 10 to 20 cm in length and is curved/ crescent in shape.
- ▶ The colour changes from green (unripe), to yellow (ripe), to black (over ripe).
- ▶ Has a thick skin that needs to be removed before eating.

221

(e)

▶ Provides a range of vitamins and minerals.
▶ Provides fibre within a diet.

Notes

1 You do not need to write out the question before answering it.
2 You only need to have the number of answers per marks given in the question. For example, (a) identify types of fruit offers two marks, so apple and pear was all that was needed.
3 If you put extra answers that are similar – for example, in (a) you wrote 'Jonathan, Braeburn, Gala', this is unlikely to have gained the two marks even though the three answers given are all types of apples.
4 If the question is an Outline, Describe or Explain, then a short sentence will be required for the answer. If you had only wrote 'Wash and cut fruit', whilst this is correct it would not have gained the two marks.
5 If you get an answer wrong and then one that is correct, you will not lose mark(s) – for example, for part (b) if you had wrote 'grapes, tomato', then you would still have gained the mark needed, for tomato.

1. NGC1 –The management of health and safety

Question 1

A manufacturing company has experienced a number of accidents that were due to poor selection and implementation of risk controls.

(a) Identify FOUR of the general principles of prevention. **(4)**
(b) Give the meaning of the term 'hierarchy of control'. **(2)**
(c) Outline how a typical hierarchy of control should be applied. **(8)**
(d) Outline the factors to be considered when selecting an appropriate risk control method. **(6)**

Answer

(a) Four general principles of prevention are:

1 the avoidance of risks;

2 the evaluation of unavoidable risks;

3 controlling hazards at source; and

4 replacing the dangerous by less or non-dangerous alternatives.

The other principles are:

5 adapting work to the individual;

6 adapting to technical progress;

7 developing a coherent prevention policy;

8 giving priority to collective over individual protective measures; and

9 giving appropriate instructions to employees.)

(b) A series of actions arranged or organised according to rank or importance designed to control risks, which are considered in order of importance, effectiveness or priority of measures. It is designed to control risks that normally begin with an extreme measure of control and end with personal protective equipment as a last resort.

(c) The first stage of the hierarchy is to eliminate the risks by either designing them out or changing the process. The next stage is the reduction of the risks by the substitution of hazardous substances with others which are less hazardous. If this were not possible, then isolation would have to be considered, using enclosures, barriers or worker segregation. The application of engineering controls such as guarding, the provision of local exhaust ventilation systems, or the use of reduced voltage systems or residual current devices would follow, as would management controls such as safe systems of work, training, job rotation and supervision, with the final control measure being the provision of personal protective equipment such as ear defenders or respiratory protective equipment.

(d) Factors to consider when selecting risk control measures include the application of the hierarchy of control. The more serious hazards may be eliminated completely – for example, by

223

avoiding working at height with the installation of a permanent working platform with stair access. In some cases, less hazardous substances or processes may be substituted, such as the use of water-based rather than oil-based paints. The control of risks by isolating them or segregating people from the hazard is an effective control measure which is used in many instances – for example, separating vehicles and pedestrians in workplaces. The rest of the hierarchy of controls may be applied in a similar way to that shown in part (c).

The evaluation of the level of risk involved, together with its likely frequency, the severity of its outcome and its extent, is another factor. Other relevant factors that should be considered include:

▶ the number and type of persons exposed to the risk;
▶ the environment in which the control is to be used;
▶ the requirements of the law and the recommendations contained in relevant standards and guidance;
▶ the existing level of competence of the persons involved, with the possible need for the provision of additional training and supervision; and
▶ the initial purchase and subsequent maintenance costs of the chosen risk control method.

Question 2

Following a reportable accident to a contractor while on an employer's premises, an investigation found that the employer had failed to provide health and safety information to the contractor. The employer was not able to demonstrate any source of competent health and safety advice.

(a) **Outline** the duties that the employer owes to the contractor under the Health and Safety at Work etc. Act 1974. **(4)**
(b) **Outline** the health and safety information that should have been provided to the contractor before work commenced. **(8)**
(c) **Outline** the factors that the employer should consider when selecting an individual to fulfil the role of health and safety practitioner. **(8)**

Answer

(a) The duties contained in Section 3 of the Health and Safety at Work (HSW) Act require an employer to ensure that persons working on its premises who are not direct employees, such as contractors, are not put at risk by the activities being carried out at the premises. Additionally, Section 4 places duties on the employer as a controller of premises, to ensure, for example, that the premises and its plant and equipment are safe and without risks to health for persons using them as a place of work.

(**Author comment**: It is possible to argue that the CDM Regulations are relevant here because all Health and Safety Regulations are made as a result of Section 15 of the HSW Act. However, in NEBOSH examinations, specific mention would be made of any Regulation that the candidates were expected to include in their answers. Hence, this question was only concerned with the specific duties included in the Act.)

(b) The health and safety information that should be provided to the contractors before work commenced would include details of any hazards in the areas where they were to work, and details of any restricted areas and those where personal protective equipment such as hearing protection would have to be worn. Information would also be required on the emergency arrangements, such as for fire and first-aid, and accident (and hazard) reporting procedures. Any general site rules – for example, for signing in and out of the site – should also be supplied, and the name and location of the designated contact person. Finally, information should be provided on any training procedures for any processes or equipment to be used by the contractor.

(c) The factors to be considered when selecting an individual to fill the role of health and safety practitioner include:

▶ previous training, qualifications and membership of professional bodies;
▶ knowledge and understanding of the role and relevant previous experience;

- ▶ understanding of the principles of risk assessment and relevant control methods;
- ▶ familiarity with relevant current legislation, standards and guidance;
- ▶ personal qualities, including ability to promote and communicate good health and safety practices;
- ▶ ability to identify problems and assess the need for action – a proactive approach;
- ▶ ability to develop and implement appropriate health and safety management strategies and evaluate their effectiveness using appropriate benchmarking data; and
- ▶ awareness of personal limitations and willingness to undertake training to rectify the deficiencies.

Question 3

Outline the general duties, under section 6 of the Health and Safety at Work etc. Act 1974, of designers, importers, manufacturers and suppliers of articles and substances for use at work to ensure that they are safe and without risk to health. **(8)**

Answer

Section 6 of the Health and Safety at Work etc. Act 1974 places an obligation on persons who design, manufacture, import or supply any article or substance for use at work to ensure, so far as is reasonably practicable, that it is safe and without risk to health. Articles must be safe when they are set, cleaned, used and maintained. Substances must be without risk to health when they are used, handled, stored or transported. Testing and examination must be carried out to ensure the required level of safety, and additionally employers should be provided with information on the safe use, dismantling and disposal of the articles and substances and given revised information should a subsequent serious risk become known. Importers have a duty to ensure articles or substances comply with the requirements of UK legislation.

The answer could be set out as follows:

1 Ensure, so far as is reasonably practicable, articles are safe and without risks to health.
2 Ensure articles are designed and constructed without risk to safety or health.
3 Undertake testing and examination.
4 Provide adequate information.
5 Provide revisions to information for serious risk.
6 Carry out research to minimize or eliminate risk.
7 Erect and/or install articles without risk to health or safety.
8 Use, handle, process, store and transport articles safely.

Question 4

(a) **Identify FIVE** common law duties that employers must fulfil to safeguard the health and safety of their employees. **(4)**
(b) **Outline** practical ways in which an employer might fulfil the four duties identified in (a). **(4)**

Answer

(a) Five common law duties that an employer must undertake are:
   ▶ provide a safe place of work, including access and egress
   ▶ provide safe plant and equipment
   ▶ provide a safe system of work
   ▶ provide safe and competent fellow employees
   ▶ provide adequate levels of supervision, information, instruction and training.

(b) A safe place of work includes items such as the structure of the building and the condition of the flooring, both of which should be sound and free of defects. There should be a safe means of access and egress to the place of work, with gangways kept clear and wide enough for traffic if it is used. Environmental factors, such as working space, lighting and heating, are also important.

Safe plant and equipment will require adequate guarding or other safety devices and regular recorded maintenance.

Safe systems of work, such as permits to work and method statements, need to be available and communicated to the workforce.

Safe and competent fellow employees can be attained through pre-selection, induction and training programmes and good supervision.

As a consequence of the fifth duty, there should be adequate levels of supervision, including mentoring and monitoring of work in progress. This duty is owed to every employee as an individual, and especially to vulnerable people, including the young and those with disabilities, and remains even when the employee may be loaned to another employer.

2. FC1 – Fire safety and risk management

Question 1

(a) Give the meaning of:
   (i) deflagration (2)
   (ii) detonation (2)
   (iii) flashpoint (2)
   (iv) auto ignition temperature (2)
   (v) upper flammable limit (UFL) (2)
   (vi) lower flammable limit (UFL). (2)
(b) Explain how a flashover may occur. (8)

Answer

(a)

Deflagration is the process of subsonic combustion whereby the flame front propagates through the un-burnt material by thermal conductivity, by which the burning material heats the next layer of un-burnt material and ignites this and continues through the layer.

Detonation is the process of combustion whereby a supersonic shock wave propagates through the material and ignites it.

Flashpoint is the lowest temperature determined under test conditions at which sufficient vapour is given off above the surface level of a substance capable of producing a flash momentarily when an external heat source is applied.

Auto-ignition is the minimum temperature at which, under specified conditions, a substance or material will ignite spontaneously and burn without the presence of any source of ignition.

Upper flammable limit is the highest concentration of vapour in air that will just support a self-propagating flame; above this limit the mixture is too rich to burn.

Lower flammable liquid is the lowest concentration of vapour in air; that will support a flame; below this limit the mixture is too lean to burn.

(b)

A flashover can occur when a fire is free burning in a room.

For this to happen, there must be a good supply of air either from the large dimension of the room or from a ventilation source.

The fire generates a high level of radiated heat that is absorbed by other materials including unburned gases in the room.

The materials and gases reach their ignition temperature and ignite even though they are not directly in contact with the flame. This giving the impression that the fire has flashed from one side of the room to the other.

Author comment: for part (a) no mark is awarded for repeating the word in the question – but two marks for the description – i.e. the marks available – will be for two different aspects of each word.

Author comment: for part (b) the answer is has been split to show EIGHT possible marks would be awarded.

Question 2

A fire has broken out in small retail shop. The fire started as a result of an electrical fault with the till and ignited some clothing on the desk.

229

Identify FOUR methods by which heat may be transferred during the fire AND describe how EACH can cause the fire to spread. (8)

Answer

▶ Direct burning – the flame from the till reaches the combustible materials and ignite them – i.e. the clothes.
▶ Conduction – the transfer of heat through solid materials involving the molecule-to-molecule transfer of heat through conducting solids such as metal beams or pipes to other parts of the shop and igniting combustible or flammable materials.
▶ Convection – the transfer of heat from a liquid or gas (i.e. air, flames or fire products) to a solid or liquid surface. Heat can be carried by rising air currents (convection) to cause a build-up of hot gases.
▶ Radiation – the emission of heat in the form of infrared radiation, which can raise temperatures of adjacent materials, for example, electric fire elements.

Author comment: four marks awarded for direct burning, conduction, convection and direct burning. The remaining four marks are given for the descriptions – one for each.

Author comment: questions 1 and 2 show examples of key words that a student should be familiar with – by working through the text book and this revision guide, you will be able to now create a list of words to learn.

Question 3

(a) Identify possible fuel sources in a small retail shop. (4)
(b) Identify possible ignition sources in a small retail shop. (4)

(a)
▶ Paper and cardboard;
▶ furniture, fixtures and fittings;
▶ wall and ceiling linings; and
▶ combustible products – e.g. clothing.

(b)

- ▶ electricity;
- ▶ illicit smoking;
- ▶ arson; and
- ▶ portable heaters.

Author comment: the question requires only an identification; therefore, a simple list is all that is required – adding additional information ('combustible products – e.g. clothing') may be helpful for clarification, even though it is an identify question.

Question 4

Outline where escape lighting system should normally cover. (8)

- ▶ At each exit door.
- ▶ On escape routes.
- ▶ At intersections of corridors.
- ▶ Outside each final exit.
- ▶ On external escape routes.
- ▶ Near to emergency escape signs.
- ▶ On stairways so that each flight receives adequate light.
- ▶ When there are changes in floor level.
- ▶ In windowless rooms.
- ▶ For toilet accommodation exceeding $8m^2$.
- ▶ Near fire-fighting equipment.
- ▶ Near fire alarm call points.
- ▶ Near to equipment that would need to be shut down in an emergency.
- ▶ Near to lifts.
- ▶ In areas in premises greater than $60m^2$.

Author comment: the above has provided 15 answers – each one is potentially worth one mark – to a maximum of eight.

✎ **Notes**

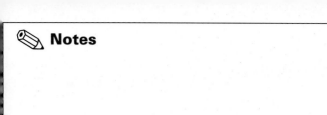

Notes

✎ **Notes**

Notes

✎ Notes